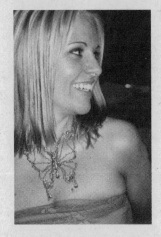

A ... b ... R ... of the hilarious and uplifting children's book *Blubberguts*. She is mother to her five-year-old son Kai (which ironically means 'food' in Maori). They live in Sydney with their pet fish, Chips, and his close personal friend, the snail, which goes by the name of Vinegar. Apart from writing AJ likes to perform corporate comedy, sing jazz, write poetry and generally have as good a time as she can without ending up in trouble of some sort (which she almost always manages to do). She also runs an online weight-loss support network, The Healthy Body Club. She speaks at many events, festivals and seminars on achieving your goals, personal motivation, health, fitness, and total wellbeing. She enjoys reading crime novels and one day dreams of writing a crime thriller that out-sells Stephen King. She does not have a problem in thinking big.

To contact AJ you can find her at ajrochester.com, healthybodyclub.com.au or on email at aj@ajrochester.com.

By the same author

Confessions of a Reformed Dieter
Blubberguts

The Lazy Girl's Guide
to Losing Weight
and Getting Fit

A.J. Rochester

BANTAM

SYDNEY AUCKLAND TORONTO NEW YORK LONDON

THE LAZY GIRL'S GUIDE TO LOSING WEIGHT AND GETTING FIT
A BANTAM BOOK

First published in Australia and New Zealand in 2005
by Bantam
This edition published in Australia and New Zealand in 2006

National Library of Australia
Cataloguing-in-Publication Entry

Rochester, A. J.
   The lazy girl's guide to losing weight and getting fit.

   ISBN 1 86325 516 8 (pbk.).

   1. Reducing diets. 2. Reducing exercises. I. Title.

   613.25

Transworld Publishers,
a division of Random House Australia Pty Ltd
20 Alfred Street, Milsons Point, NSW 2061
http://www.randomhouse.com.au

Random House New Zealand Limited
18 Poland Road, Glenfield, Auckland

Transworld Publishers,
a division of The Random House Group Ltd
61–63 Uxbridge Road, Ealing, London W5 5SA

Random House Inc
1745 Broadway, New York, New York 10036

Typeset by Midland Typesetters, Australia
Printed and bound by Griffin Press, Netley, South Australia

¹0 9 8 7 6 5 4 3 2 1

For my beautiful goddaughter, Minna-Moo.
The depth of your talent astounds me.
Dare to be the very best that you can be.
You truly are a star.
Love you,
Aunty Lu-Lu

Warning!

This is not a diet book. There are no secrets to instant-aneous weight loss. This is an easy to follow guide to changing your life for the better and losing weight along the way.

To all those wanting to take that brave step towards learning to love yourself, I truly wish you the very best of luck!

Contents

Foreword

When I got my dream job on a magazine, one of my first tasks was to compile the annual 'Diet Special'. This involved scouring old issues of the magazine and picking out the diets that made the biggest promises: i.e., the largest weight loss in the shortest time.

Some of these corkers included the 'Honey and Wheatgerm Diet' and my personal fave, the 'Drop-A-Dress-Size-By-Saturday Diet'. Having struggled with my own body image demons through my teens and knowing loads of girls with eating disorders, I knew instinctively that diets were not the answer. Lord knows I'd tried enough of them and all they did was make me obsess about whichever food that particular diet banned (which, in the case of the 'Drop-A-Dress-Size-By-Saturday Diet', was pretty much everything) and trigger a post-deprivation pig-out.

Five years later, when I became an editor myself, I swore that I would use my new power for good, not evil. The first thing I did was to ban diets, and the second thing I did was to start using models of all sizes and shapes. I felt passionately that skinny, tall, white girls with blonde hair shouldn't be the only type of sexy female portrayed in the media. I wanted women of all sizes to feel positive about their bodies, and seeing those bodies reflected on the pages of a glossy women's magazine was, I felt, a vital step. I danced on this particular soapbox for several years and tried to encourage more of my sister editors to take a similar approach, instead of using human coat hangers on every page.

A few years into my crusade, I was sent a book called *Confessions of a Reformed Dieter*. I binge-read it in one night and recognised so much of myself and my friends on every page. It was a real *ka-ching* moment for me and it changed my approach to food and exercise in my own life and in my magazines.

I emailed the author, AJ Rochester, immediately and threw my media weight behind helping her get as many people as possible to buy her book. Why? Because in charting her own journey with such brutal honesty, AJ made women feel like they weren't alone – because no matter how fat or thin you are, body image hell is a very lonely, private battle. More importantly, she simplified the enormous complexity of weight loss into three simple parts: what you eat, what you do and what you feel.

To me, this was the key. If you don't understand why you are eating too much, or too little, then you can't expect to achieve a healthy weight. Sitting on the couch eating a packet of biscuits in one night is not about honouring your body or celebrating your right to eat chocolate. It is not empowering. It's as abusive to your body as starving it or throwing up your dinner. That's why AJ's book was such a gift to every woman, large or small, who has found herself on the food/emotional roller coaster and who would very much like to get off and find her happy weight.

The Lazy Girl's Guide to Losing Weight and Getting Fit is just as tasty. Recognising aspects of your own body battles in *Confessions of a Reformed Dieter* is the first part of winning the war. The second part comes with the very detailed advice, instruction and support that AJ has shared in this wonderful book. This is not a diet book. It's a hundred times better because it is real and life-changing. Tell your friends about it. Tell your mum. Spread the love.

Mia Freedman
Editor-In-Chief, *Cosmopolitan, Cleo, Dolly*

Introduction – Shazam!

Let's start by getting honest with each other. How many times in the last month have you promised yourself that tomorrow was definitely going to be the start of your brand new diet? Once? Twice? Eight times? I bet you've been doing it all your life. Well, let me tell you the first thing you need to know: *diets don't work.* In fact, I believe that dieting makes you fat. Every diet I ever went on made me fatter, unhappier and totally convinced I would never be a success.

That was, until the day I decided to change the way I lived my life. One year later I wound up eight dress sizes smaller. Interestingly, not once did I mention the word 'diet'. Now let me tell you some things about myself: if there is a shortcut, or any way to cheat, then I will. If there is any way I can eat the food I love – comfort food and junk – without putting on weight, then I will. If there is a way to lose weight without giving up champagne then that is the way for me. I am the laziest girl in the world – no contest – and if I can do it, anyone can. No excuses.

This book will show you how to lose that excess weight without pills, shakes, wraps, cabbage soup or liposuction. And the best thing is that you can have your cake and eat it too, sometimes.

Now for the bad news: put that piece of chocolate down and repeat after me: 'I hereby promise to give up chocolate, cheesecake, Pluto Pups, hot chips, pizza, beer, champagne . . . in fact I'll just stop eating everything I love and become a perfect food and exercise angel and will be thin, happy and beating the opposite sex off with a cattle prod in no time at all.'

Snore . . . You don't actually believe that, do you?

If you do, go back to pigging out on chocolate and hot dogs 'cause if you are anything like me, you know nothing like that will ever happen. You can't give up *everything* just to lose weight. Well, you can, but how boring would you be? For me, life just wouldn't be the same without my weekly champagne and Keanu Reeves film fests. OK, I could possibly give up Keanu, but not the champers. At least, not forever.

If you want to live your life to the fullest, treat yourself well and eat the food you love while losing weight and getting fit, healthy and happy, follow me. Hang on, I'm sure I told you to put that piece of chocolate down. Remember that (despite popular belief among my fellow fatties) just because no one is watching you eat that contraband doesn't mean there aren't any calories in it. Now repeat after me:

> *I commit to being the very best that I can be. I deserve to love, be loved and most importantly of all, I deserve to love myself. I deserve a healthy body and I will never give up on myself, no matter what happens, and I promise to do whatever it takes to make it happen. Today is the first day of the rest of my life. Shazam!*

This is your new mantra or pledge to yourself. Repeat it every time you feel like giving up, or after every setback you have (and you will have them). Dust the cake crumbs from your mouth and get right back on that little weight-loss horsey – it's going to keep you heading in a forward direction. All the way to I-know-you-want-me-but-you-can't-have-me Land.

Warning: This next bit may hurt but compare it to trying to squeeze yourself into a sexy size 10 bikini in a brightly-lit change room, two weeks before summer. Oh, the pain.

Go straight to your fridge and cupboard (do not pass the cookie jar, do not collect 200 calories). Throw out all the biscuits, chips, lollies, ice-cream, frozen food, junk food, packet food and deep-fried, reheat, do-it-yourself, heart-attack-in-a box food items. I repeat, throw it all out – *don't* go making yourself one last meal. If you cook roast pork followed by chocolate pudding with ice cream and five bottles of wine just because you'll be going 'without' for the next few months, you'll end up three kilos heavier than you were before you started. This isn't a diet, remember, it's a healthy eating plan, a new way to live your life. There is no such thing as one last meal or one last treat. You are *not* going without, I promise you. Prohibition doesn't work. You *will* still have your favourite foods, you *will* still have a drink, and you *will* still treat yourself with chocolate, or whatever else your vice is, but *just not every day*. And believe me when I tell you: you'll discover *new* favourite foods.

Also, if you think that you have to wait for the beginning of the week or the first of the month or after your sexy weekend away to start eating healthily, then you have got it all wrong. That's just an excuse for not actually doing this. Hello?! I've heard them all before – I'm sure I invented at least half of the excuses ever used.

Either you're with me or you're not – and if you're not then I guess I won't be seeing you on the beach next summer, unless Greenpeace are pushing you back out to sea. And don't bother filling out an organ donor card 'cause no one's going to want your heart after you're finished with it. Harsh, aren't I? Well, to be totally honest, if you really don't want to change your life, nothing I say will make a difference.

If you're with me, your new life starts *now*. Not tomorrow, not next week, or next month, or New Year's Day or three months before your birthday . . . right now. The very next meal you have will be healthier and I promise, you'll feel just a little bit better about yourself – not because you weigh a kilo less, but because you are in control and looking after yourself.

Now, say the pledge again and try to mean it:

I commit to being the very best that I can be. I deserve to love, be loved and most importantly of all, to love myself. I deserve a healthy body and I will never give up on myself, no matter what happens, and I promise to do whatever it takes to make it happen. Today is the first day of the rest of my life. Shazam!

I know you don't really believe it, but one day you will. I promise.

1

A Brief, Ancient History of Me

Once upon a time I was fat. Really fat. I was so fat my bum had its own postcode. My breasts were so big that when I went to parties I was the booby prize. I didn't have bras, I had aircraft hangars. I had more chins than a Chinese phone book. I was a very big girl.

It was not uncommon for me to down a large BBQ Meat Lover's pizza, six deep-fried chicken wings, a whole garlic bread and cheesecake for dinner, followed by two bottles of wine, and end up with the midnight munchies where it would start all over again. And just in case you think I hadn't made enough of a pig of myself I was also guilty of ordering extra packets of ranch dressing (for the chicken wings) and smothering it on top of the pizza. I had an eating disorder (oh really?) and it wasn't until I accepted that eating for five was perhaps not the norm that I started to get well on the inside, outside and backside.

I hated myself and treated myself with absolutely no respect. I felt trapped, desperately unhappy, out of control and most of the time I wished I was dead.

Now, here's the thing: I didn't hate myself for being *fat* – I don't love myself any more now because I'm not fat – I hated being out of control; I hated the fact that I was killing myself slowly with food; I hated that I had stopped participating in life because I just didn't love myself enough. I hated myself because I was hiding in my fat and only half living my life. Now I know I never loved myself, not even when I was younger, thinner and 'prettier'. My body was a reflection of what I felt on the inside. I carried so much pain and grief, and had been subjected to so much abuse, that I simply continued that behaviour in whatever form it took: binge drinking, drug-taking, under-eating, over-eating – all of which eventually led me to become obese.

So, you ask, how did all this happen? Well, you could say I had a few [insert theme from *Psycho*] issues. Loosely translated, I was a walking, talking basket case. But not always . . .

I was born in Sydney on 17 April, 1969. My birth mother was an up and coming model, single and, like most pregnant unmarried mothers, was coerced into giving up her child (me) to a much more socially suitable, Anglo Saxon *married* couple. They had already adopted a boy two years older than me. We lived a normal, middle class existence in the suburbs of Sydney. I had a very active life, keeping fit and busy with ballet, physical culture, swimming, tennis and riding my bike anywhere I could get away with. One day, just after my eighth birthday, my father announced that we were moving to the country. He was following his life-long dream and was going to become a farmer. He assured us it would be the best time of our lives.

But life was not the fairy tale my father had promised. A school teacher molested me, and things weren't terrific at home. My parents split up when I was sixteen and I took the very first bus back to Sydney as quickly as I could. Then, in my late teens, I was raped by someone I thought I could trust. After years of longing to know my origins, I finally found my birth mother (which didn't do much for my relationship with my adopted mother). In a strange twist of fate, I had been working in my mother's theatre restaurant for a year without knowing who she was.

I remember my boyfriend at the time joking that her first name was the same as my mum's, and that she could actually be my mum. I laughed it off, saying she was too young. What a shock it was to find that she was indeed the woman I had been longing to know my entire life. Less than a year later I lost her to a tragic and senseless death. I was truly alone and felt totally abandoned and betrayed. After losing my birth mother for the second time I think I just gave up on myself – nobody loved me so why should I bother? It was one of the saddest, loneliest times of my life and I am surprised I survived it.

I tracked down my birth father, who had married and had four other children, but I didn't find any answers and I subsequently found myself feeling rejected once more. I felt as if I would never be good enough and through my twenties I struggled through abusive relationships, and turned to drugs and alcohol. I was a walking, talking disaster zone.

I never learned to love and nurture myself – all I really knew was abuse and lack of respect. When I left home I just continued that cycle of abuse, first by developing anorexia and then bulimia. After collapsing from malnutrition, and being told by a nurse that I was going to die if I didn't start eating properly and stop poisoning my underweight body with laxatives, I then attempted to eat myself to death. It wasn't pretty and, even though I used to tell myself that one day I was going to get healthy, I'm not sure I ever really believed it, deep down. To me it seemed like an impossible dream. It was what other people did. Oprah got fit – I was never going to be good enough to do that. My mantra was that I was a complete failure and could never take control of my life.

Despite labelling myself a failure, and weighing a

whopping 109 kilograms, I still managed to carve out a fairly decent career in comedy, both in Australia and overseas. I worked on cruise ships, then in the corporate scene, got a decent amount of gigs in film, TV and radio, developed a reasonable reputation as a writer and spoken word artist (a fancy name for performance poet), and co-hosted the very successful SBS TV series *Mum's the Word*. Being big meant I was considered a 'minority' in TV terms, which meant I was perfect for SBS, despite being Anglo Saxon!

Anyway, wanting to promote myself as the next big thing (ha ha) in TV (wanting my own sketch comedy show), I decided to try to make the best, or the breast, of my best *ass*ets (or the best of my breast assets?). There was only ever one fat girl on each drama or comedy, and I wanted to be it. I planned a publicity stunt and declared 'National Flesh is Best Day' staging a huge demonstration at Sydney Town Hall. We had belly dancers, clowns, body painters, waifs begging for chocolate and a whole host of people carrying placards with catchy slogans like 'I shop at Big Flesh', 'Don't put a fatwah on me', 'I'm Fat-tastic' and 'My Boobs and Chest are Rubenesque'. We had petitions demanding bigger seating in planes, fairer sizing in the clothing industry and more real women (like me!) on TV.

As a great day out it was an absolute hoot, but as a publicity stunt it was a big fat disaster, pardon the pun. Only one film crew showed up and they were from The Lifestyle Channel on Foxtel and were doing a documentary on *obesity*. That was it. Not another camera in sight. The only person interested in filming me was there because I was not only fat, but *obese*. Incredibly, I had never applied that terrible word to my own idea of myself. My world came crashing down … I was so busy calling myself a goddess I didn't realise I had been deceiving myself.

That night I cried myself to sleep. I was a single mother only just past thirty and at great risk of actually dying from my ballooning weight. I didn't want to die, and I certainly didn't want to die from being too fat. Coming to that realisation was my turning point. Every ex-fat chick has had one and every fat chick knows that one day she will have one. That was mine; the point of no return. The day that I decided to change the way I lived my life – forever.

The producer of the program had made an appointment with me to do a full-length interview. There was no way I was going to go on the record saying I was fat, proud of it and happy to stay that way. I knew my eating habits were terrible, I knew my health was an issue (I couldn't walk up a flight of stairs without feeling as though I was having a heart attack), and if I was ever going to do something about it then this was the time – enough was enough. I was prepared to do whatever I needed to take control of my life.

By the time the producer turned up I had hatched a plan. I wasn't sure I'd be able to complete it but I was going to give it my best shot.

I got myself a personal trainer I called Crusher, a shrink I called Dr Nutcase and a nutritionist I named Beansprout. I learned how, what and when to eat, trained myself to move, broke my leg two weeks into my 'diet', ended up in a wheelchair, continued to exercise, started swimming, and discovered aquarobics. When I was out of the wheelchair I took up walking (this time with a walking stick and a limp), was told I would never run, then took up running and completed the City to Surf (a 14 kilometre fun run), joined a women's soccer team, dealt with the demons having a party in my head, gave up my addiction to fast food and chocolate (I'm still working on the addiction to alcohol!), and somewhere in the mix I managed to lose over 45 kilos. Just like that. Actually, it wasn't just like that. It was the hardest thing I have ever done, and yet it was easier and quicker than I imagined it would be. Time passes quickly when you are focused. One minute you're complaining that you can't buy jeans in your size, and the next you're ranting about how size 12 jeans are just too big.

Anyway, the producer and I agreed to put a camera in my house and I did weekly video diary updates and filmed whenever I had a melt down or crack up (which was pretty much every second day in the beginning). Those video diary updates later became the foundation for the very popular documentary *Larger Than Life* and still airs regularly on the Lifestyle Channel on Foxtel.

On a whim I decided to record the whole process in print as well: warts and all. I've kept diaries for most of my life, but this one became my safe haven and in my darkest hours it was my closest friend. It was the only place I could admit to how much I actually ate; it was the only place I could pour out all that was in my heart. My diary was where I went to get things straight in my head.

At first I was devastated at just how much I had to deal with to lose the weight I had been carrying around for so long. I wasn't just mildly overweight – I was morbidly obese. I'm not sure whether I had more fat than emotional baggage, but they were both bloody heavy and very difficult to deal with. I couldn't believe how many of my friends and family members were unable to support me; and also how many actually tried to sabotage me. But I soldiered on, determined to change my life for the better. I wrote it all down, everything I learned, all my trials, triumphs and tribulations. I did whatever Crusher, Nutcase and Bean-sprout told me, I committed to the final outcome and eventually managed to shave an entire person off my body.

That diary became my book, *Confessions of a Reformed*

Dieter, and before I knew it, the girl who was once the fast food queen somehow became a very reluctant 'dieting' queen (who truly believes diets don't work). Little did I know the book would be a bestseller and end up being sold around the world. If I'd known that I might not have admitted I had become so fat I could no longer reach around to wipe my bum. *Sigh*. Oh, for the power to predict the future!

The other thing I didn't plan for was the thousands of emails I received from (mostly) women saying, 'Oh my god, that is my life! It's exactly how I feel and what I have done to myself for most of my life.' How could so many women feel the way I did? I had always felt so totally isolated within my eating disorder and self-hatred. How could there be so many women who hated themselves as much as me, and felt like I did – near suicidal – because their eating was way out of control? After so many women begged me to get involved in helping them change their lives and asking me what exactly I did to get to my goal, I finally decided to do something about it.

I started my own weight loss/personal training/dietary advice, support and motivation service called The Healthy Body Club. I advise people wanting to lose weight and am constantly surprised by just how little they know about how to get fit and change their life. I never imagined I would be doing this, but the universe has many plans and somehow destiny pulls you in a way you can never imagine. But then, I have always been slightly megalomaniacal. And it just seems completely selfish to know what to do and to not share it with everyone else!

It's been such a joy to see women transform their lives. At first they are exhausted and devastated from trying to lose weight for months, or even years, on end and having had absolutely no success – or have had a little success and have put it all, and more, back on. Very slowly I take them through the process . . . and wham, bam, thank-you ma'am, they start to lose weight – all of them averaging about a kilo a week, just as I did. There are no big secrets, special shakes or magic little pills, and the formula is quite simple and allows you to have the things you want, and enable you to live your life as well. And it works on even the toughest of my clients . . . and not once do we utter the 'D' word. It's true: diets don't work.

Since my book *Confessions* was published the most common email of all has been, 'Thanks heaps, really inspiring, but how *exactly* did you do it?' After so many emails pleading with me to share my 'secrets' I couldn't really keep it all to myself. The secret is that I had to relearn the way I lived, moved, ate, thought and felt about myself. Once I did that the weight loss was easy.

If you do the work on the inside, the outside will follow.

This book is a record of everything I have learned about losing weight, getting healthy and learning to love yourself. But you won't find any fantastical weight loss secrets here. What you *will* find are all the techniques I used to help me lose weight. Sorting out the calories and fat content was the easy part; working out why I craved bad food, and found ways to trick myself into eating well, was what *really* helped me shave the equivalent of Calista Flockhart off my body.

But first, before you read on, there is one thing I must clarify. Losing weight and becoming a healthy size 12 *did not* make me happy – *getting healthy* made me happy. If you think losing X amount of dress sizes or kilos will solve all your problems, you have failed before you've even started because good health and happiness begins within. Size has nothing to do with it.

Sure, being healthy makes me happy, possibly extends my

life (but I may die in an horrific aeroplane crash next week, who knows?), and enables me to conduct a healthier, more physically active life with my beautiful son Kai, but being happy is what keeps me alive and loving and respecting myself. Those things, ironically, also keep me healthy. I do not advocate the be-a-size-10-and-find-ultimate-happiness ideology. That is a myth manufactured by the diet industry. You have to get happy and healthy on the inside before you can even begin on the outside. And you *can* be a size 14 or a size 16 – as long as you are happy and more importantly, healthy.

Now, for all those people saying, 'There are plenty of people who are fat and happy.' You're right, but the reality is that being overweight is *not* healthy. If you are fat and happy and content to stay that way then this is not the book for you. I wish you all the best and hope you live a long and industrious life despite the heart transplant you'll be having when you turn forty. This book is for those who are not happy with the way they are, for those who know they deserve more, who want to be able to fit into the swings at the park, who want to be able to run for the bus without having a heart attack, and for those who want to walk into a shop without being directed to the 'You'll need a dancing hippo, fifteen clowns, a really small car and a ringmaster with that dress' department, otherwise known as the plus size section of Kmart. Ugh!

With that little gem in mind, follow me.

Quick Quiz

1. When you need new clothes you:
   a) Shop at Tent City.
   b) Stay away from the mall and drag out your old muu muus, which are starting to feel too tight.
   c) Slip on those size 8 Calvin Kleins you've had your eye on and breeze out the door.

2. Your friends invite you to the beach but:
   a) Only because your shadow stops them from getting too much sun.
   b) You refuse, not wanting to be stalked by Mimi McPherson's whale watching crew.
   c) You are entering Miss Indy and will be too busy strutting around town in a bikini and high heels, being chased by the paparazzi.

3. When feeling peckish:
   a) You eat at Maccas because you are a gold member customer for having eaten there so often, and Ronald McDonald personally presented you with a shares portfolio thanking you for your patronage.
   b) You call Dial-a-Dumpster and get them to stop off at Pizza Hut.
   c) You dine on carrot sticks, celery and your favourite meal of all – fresh air.

Mostly a: You need to read this book and you know it. You are sick to death of never having anything to wear, you don't want to break any more chairs and you no longer want your beautician to cringe fearfully every time you climb up on her table to have your eyebrows shaped. Well done. It is time to change your life.

Mostly b: Well, you're certainly ready to read this book but I'm not sure you'll live long enough to finish it. Get your fat arse moving, girl. What are you waiting for? Jesus to come back as a Pluto Pup?

Mostly c: As my son Kai would say, 'You're crackin' jokes.' Get outta here.

2

Getting Started

You are now entering The Alfalfa Zone

'The cheapest form of exercise you can do is exercise
mind over platter.'
Unknown

If you are truly ready to stop hating yourself, and are willing
to do whatever it takes to break the cycle of abusing yourself
with food, there are a couple of things I need to tell you
before you read on.

The first is that it won't be easy. There are some shortcuts
but in all honesty, changing a lifetime of habits takes time,
effort and great commitment. No one else can do this for
you; only you can save yourself. It *will* be hard. However, the
second thing you need to know is that it will actually be
easier than you ever imagined.

Let me put it this way: do you know how hard it is to eat a
whole BBQ Meat Lover's pizza, six deep fried chicken wings
and a garlic bread followed by a whole chocolate cheesecake
and still respect yourself in the morning? It's damn hard.
Believe me when I say it is easier to just grab a piece of fruit
and a tub of yoghurt (not to mention being a hell of a lot cheaper).

When I first started on my journey I remember watching
the clock tick, salivating and fantasising about food until it
was time for my next meal. I found myself obsessing about
food more than I thought possible. I remember crying
because I thought I'd never eat pizza or Pluto Pups ever again.

I remember feeling like a freak and wanting to be normal, but not believing it was possible, and wondering if I would ever achieve what seemed to be an unreachable dream. I wanted to be in control, not crumble at the whim of my food addictions, be strong, fit and not blame my fat for the cause of all my unhappiness. And I wanted to look and feel great.

Eventually, with persistence, a few hundred setbacks and a hell of a lot of work, time passed, things changed and 45 kilos lighter I realised that it wasn't anywhere near as impossible as I thought it would be. Time flies, believe me, much faster than you think. The women who join my weight loss club have had enough. They have been in the gym and on the dieting treadmill for years and are totally convinced that a healthy body is completely unattainable for them.

But it *is* possible – even for the laziest and most hopeless of cases. I was exactly that – bloody hopeless. I couldn't even run to the Mr. Whippy van, and I wanted to! I thought that losing weight went hand in hand with going without, and having to work too hard for very little reward or success. I also thought it should happen overnight. This is one of the greatest myths we need to break down. It doesn't take two weeks for you to put a lot of weight on, so why expect it all to come off in such an unreasonable time frame?

The healthiest way to lose weight is to take it easy, and do it slowly so that you learn new habits that are sustainable for the rest of your life. Losing a half to one kilo a week at the most is the most achievable, and the best for your body *and* your brain. Any more than that is unhealthy.

Surely the greatest reward is a healthy, happier, longer life? I say, give it a good six months. Do the very best that you can, make all the changes (or as many as you can cope with at any given time), be as honest as you can and work as hard as it is possible for you to work (while allowing yourself to cheat just a little bit) and see how much of a difference that small amount of time can make. Because compared to all the years you have been unhappy with yourself (and all the fashions you have missed) six months isn't such a big commitment, is it?

But whatever your time frame is, the weight will go if you are committed to it going. You may work out that it will take twelve months to reach your goal weight. Some lucky people may only need three or four months. It might take you two or three years. Whatever it is, you have the rest of your life to enjoy it. Don't rush!

Think about how many years have passed since you decided for the millionth time that you were no longer going to be overweight. Time has a funny habit of passing. You have to remember that this is an investment in the rest of your life, so take your time and enjoy the ride. It *will* be bumpy, but better that than your thighs!

The other thing you need to know is that there will be times when you *do* 'fail'. Remember, though, that without 'failing' we would never learn. None of us is perfect. I can't tell you how many times I crumbled and ended up devouring a Pluto Pup and fries followed by an entire block of Fruit 'n' Nut chocolate (and it still happens occasionally, but now only about once a year). As long as the next meal is a healthy one, and the next one, and the next one after that, the blowout may have been one step backwards, but ultimately you've taken three steps forward. No matter how long it takes, *you will* eventually end up in front!

Now, let's get this party started.

1. Get ready

Check your health with your doctor. Let them know what you are about to do and have your blood pressure, cholesterol, blood sugar and thyroid levels checked. Once you get the all clear, you are ready to change your life for the better.

2. Get clean – go through your cupboards

You didn't throw all that food away, did you? What are you waiting for? The second coming? If you keep stuffing your face with those hot chips then you won't be around to see the second coming, so just do it. While you're at it you may as well get rid of your alcohol too – wrap it up and give it to your neighbour. Look at it this way: the more they drink, the better you look, so it's not really wasting it, is it? Remember this is not forever, just until you start to see some improvements; but if you keep it around till then, you won't see any changes soon.

Temptation is your worst enemy. When you are craving those crispy little dim sims you keep in the freezer for that special occasion, or want to drown your lack of Keanu's (sorrows) in a bottle of vodka (or is that just me?) those little fatty balls of pseudo happiness are just too easy to access in that moment of weakness. A lot of people say they don't have the willpower to lose weight. I used to think that one day I would wake up and suddenly have that special power which would finally help me make the changes I needed in my life. Well, it doesn't happen. Willpower actually has nothing to do with it. Cravings are cravings and there's not a lot anyone can do about them except make them difficult to satisfy. Hence, get rid of the dim sims and make your house safe. Every single person in the world has cravings, no matter how 'perfect' they may seem to be. Cravings are generally temporary and pass after you have satisfied yourself in another way. I'll talk to you more about how to deal with cravings successfully a little later on.

3. Get safe – take control of your environment

It's not just your house you need to make free from rubbish food. You need a safe work environment as well. If you have co-workers who buy you treats or supply morning tea you need to ask them not to include you, or, if they do, ask them to buy some healthy choices (or you'll sue their asses off for bodily abuse!). You might even inspire everyone else to get healthy.

Put a big bowl of fresh fruit next to the biscuit tin. That way you can train yourself to make a healthy choice. Notice that I said 'train'. Good health is something you learn, not something that is delivered in a packet – just add water and an empty bank account. You need to teach yourself what, how and when to eat.

Now, this next piece of advice is non-negotiable: *always* have water on hand. Chill it so it's nice to drink. If you've been drinking sweet drinks for a long time then water may not satisfy you at first, so use diet cordial or a squeeze of lemon or lime. Your taste buds will hate you at first but they will adapt. It should take a couple of weeks, but after that you'll be OK. Trust me, I'm adopted. It does take some getting used to but so does having to wear your skirt with the zip undone because your stomach arrives five minutes before you do. You make the choice.

Let your friends and family know what you are doing and enlist their support. Ask them not to bring junk food into your house. Ask them not to give you chocolate or alcohol as a gift, even if you do have a family like mine and you need to drink to avoid murdering them. If they can't support you in this you should really start to question their motives.

Unfortunately, one of the realities of making enormous changes is that some people may not want you to change.

Some people like you the way you are because it makes them feel better about themselves. One of the confronting things about no longer living your life dysfunctionally is that the other dysfunctional people in your life have to face up to, or refuse to accept, reality themselves. All *you* need to do is decide to get healthy and live your life the very best way you can. People will either be with you, or they will fall by the wayside. Remember, though, you will not only survive, but you will thrive as well.

If you attend any mothers' groups or meet friends regularly for a coffee take something healthy to eat instead of ordering up big on the chocolate cake (I do this with Betty Crocker Low Fat Fudge Brownies – individually wrapped).

Don't buy junk food regularly for your kids. Not only will you be tempted to buy it for yourself but you'll probably end up having a few chips here, a couple of nuggets there (and they do add up). And why on earth would you want to make your kids fat? Not only are you reducing their chances at leading a healthy and happy life but you're teaching them the wrong message about food and eating well. If you're going to treat the kids, keep aside the money you would spend on junk and in four weeks time let them spend that money on whatever they want in a toy shop. I can tell you now that after one spree in that toy shop they won't feel like they're missing out.

4. Get honest and gather evidence

Next step – take a photo of yourself. Let it all hang out and record your 'former' self forever. You're going to need it because in a period of time it will be your 'before' photo. You will *never* look like this again. I know you'd rather weigh yourself down with a billion chocolate bars and throw yourself into a very deep lake of maple syrup than actually see yourself semi-naked, but you will need this photo when you are about half-way through your weight loss and hit the dreaded plateau. When you do, you dig out this photo and remind yourself just how far you have come.

When I was half-way through my weight loss, I went home for Christmas, proud that I had shed 23 kilos (a little more weight than that of my five-year-old). My dad greeted me with the words, 'You might have lost a little around your face', and my grandmother said, 'How much weight do you reckon you've lost? You're kidding yourself if you've lost six.' Those comments sent me into a deep, downward spiral. It wasn't until my step-mum showed me a photo of myself taken twelve months earlier that I realised I had done an amazing job and nothing or no one would stop me from reaching my goal.

While we're on the honesty train you should weigh and measure yourself as well. I know you don't want to. Ignorance is bliss, isn't it? Actually, it's not. Finding out what you weigh could be what actually motivates you. I was 109 kilos! When I figured out that, in all probability, the Goodyear Blimps I called my breasts weighed 5 kilos each I was more than happy to put the Pluto Pups down. When you've figured out how much you weigh, you'll need to figure out how much weight you need or want to lose, and I talk about this a bit later in the next chapter.

Every time you weigh yourself you need to wear the same clothes, and use the same scales. Different sets of scales differ and you don't want to set yourself up for feelings of failure just because you weigh in on somebody else's scales. You also need to weigh yourself at the same time of the day. You weigh more at night so you are better off weighing in first thing in the morning. And here's the big one: only weigh yourself once a week. Don't do it every day – it just messes with your head. Also, never weigh yourself when you have your period – wait till the next week. At this time of the month you retain fluid and can weigh up to *3 kilos* heavier! I know I do.

When doing your measurements you need to measure your neck, chest, waist, wrist, bicep (that's your upper arm), hips and thigh. There's a handy chart to use on page 279. I know the idea of measuring your neck seems strange but I lost 13 cm off mine, so go figure. The reason why you measure yourself is because, sometimes, you might not have lost any weight according to the scales, but your body shape may still be changing. If you are walking, running, swimming or working out at a gym you will be building muscle and muscle is actually denser, or heavier, than fat. Sometimes the scales may not tell the real story. The added bonus about muscle is that it burns fat just by being there – so when you gain muscle you become a fat-burning machine. How good is that?

Next, open your wardrobe and dig out something lovely or sexy that doesn't fit you any more. Or, if you're like me, find something you bought that you couldn't quite fit into because you were definitely going on a diet the very next day. Try it on for size, even if it means lying on the floor and pushing your belly in the same way you would stuff a Christmas turkey. In a little while your item of choice will glide effortlessly over your hips, harp music will play in the background and gorgeous naked men will spring out from behind the curtains to fan you with palm fronds and feed you grapes. Well, perhaps not the harps, grapes and spunks bit but you'll definitely be able to fit into your pants.

It's a great way to monitor your progress. Once again, you

may find that, from time to time, you haven't lost weight on the scales but that item of clothing is looser. One day it will actually fit you – and sooner than you think. It's a wonderful incentive. As your hard work pays off, having something sexy that almost fits, and then fits you perfectly, means you can see it (and feel it) in real terms.

For those of you like me, you may have had thinner days, so dig out a photo of yourself from that time and put it somewhere to remind you of your goal. If it was fifteen years ago and you've had twenty kids since then it may not be realistic to get back to *exactly* that weight. I would rather be a healthy size 12 than struggle to stay a tiny size 10 – I like my food and champers far too much. You just have to decide what you want out of life. But focusing on a healthier you and knowing you were that size once before can really motivate you to get out of bed that little bit earlier each day – enough to go for that walk that will make all the difference.

And now to the most important thing of all: the food diary (your copy is on page 280). You just don't know how much rubbish you eat until you start to write it all down. I talk about this in much more detail later but you will be surprised to see just how much unhealthy food and drink you are consuming. I know from experience that becoming obese demanded a considerable commitment to bad food – and it's not easy eating eight fish finger sandwiches in one sitting! It's simply amazing how focused the food diary can keep you.

It's interesting how it works: the process of recording what you eat suddenly helps you want to make better choices. Once you start being honest about what you eat you take great steps towards living a healthier life. You can also look back over a day or a week and see where you could have made a healthier choice, then promise to implement it next time. You can also add up your fat and calorie intakes and work out how much you need to cut it down to get into weight-loss mode. Remember, keeping a food diary is not negotiable. You *have* to do it.

5. Get help

Now that you have made the decision to change your life, you need to know that, first, it is a life-long decision, and second, that you will be changing both your eating *and* emotional habits. This brings me to my Dr Nutcase: I enlisted the help of a shrink who specialises in eating disorders. I believe anyone who can drag me away from BBQ Meat Lover's pizzas long enough to learn to live healthily and ultimately love myself has to be doing something right.

Most of the people who contact me know they have an eating disorder. It can manifest itself in many ways – over-eating, under-eating, eating the wrong food, over-exercising, vomiting, abusing themselves with laxatives or a combination of any, or all of these. I can't say enough for the benefits of getting a professional to help you break those very vicious cycles. I dealt with a lot of issues I had about food, eating and self-image, and I will share with you what I have learned in this book, but only you can discover why you treat yourself the way you do. Everyone is different, and you need to find out what drives you to do the things you do, and what will personally work for you.

I also used to think that when I finally got to a certain weight I'd be happy. But as my weight dropped – first to 99 kilos, then 89, then 79, then 69, and then 64 – Dr Nutcase pointed out that it might not matter what weight I was; the issue could be that I was just generally very unhappy.

We figured out together that the weight was just an excuse. When I accepted that and began to work on what was really making me unhappy, my weight didn't seem so important – and yet it continued to drop off. I learned to work on being happy rather than using my fat as an excuse for my emotional state. Once I did that, I naturally ate healthier food and took better care of myself. It was a not-so-vicious cycle that worked very effectively.

There are many professionals around who can help you. To see a psychiatrist you need to get a referral from your doctor. You can book an appointment with a psychologist of your choice whenever you like but there is no Medicare rebate on their services. There are also support groups such as Overeaters Anonymous and the Eating Disorders Foundation (see the Contacts section). Outpatient services at hospitals are also easily accessed and don't forget the net – there are plenty of sites that offer support, guidance and sometimes even incentives such as personal training on-line, prizes, or even cash for weight loss.

If you aren't quite ready for counselling then enlist the help of a friend. Find someone who will listen to and support you; someone you trust enough to ring and tell them you could murder your grandmother for a Meat Lover's pizza. Make sure they are someone *you* will listen to, as well. Get them to remind you of your goals in your moment of weakness. Get them to remind you to do your pledge and think about your new body. Let them know how you are feeling and what you are going through. And listen to them when they use a megaphone to tell you to back away from the fridge and go for a walk. I ring my friend Zoe. I say, 'Give me a pep talk about exercise or eating healthily.' She does, and I hang up, once more focused on what I want to achieve.

Weight Watchers is a good place to find support. There is safety in numbers, and they have excellent magazines and books with inspirational stories, tips and advice, and have recently introduced the issue of emotional eating into their program.

Major weight loss can be a difficult emotional journey and you are no less a person for admitting you need help. If you are abusing food and your body you will need some form of professional assistance to help you create new habits. And remember, if you don't like the first thing you try then shop around and find something or someone that does work for you.

Remember, though, that at some point the buck stops with you. You have to take responsibility for the way you are and commit yourself to change. Only then will it all fall into place.

6. Get real

Now, set yourself some goals. No, you can't include David Beckham or Jude Law in them, they're mine! Seriously, make them realistic and achievable, and write them down. Make a personal contract with yourself – and sign it.

If you need to lose 20 kilos then aim for 10 and deal with the other 10 when you get there. If you need to lose 50 kilos, concentrate on the first 20 and break that down to 5 at a time. Focusing on achievable goals is the foundation rule for my health club. Forty-five kilos seemed impossible to me but 5 each time was do-able. If I was focused, losing 5 kilos would take me about five weeks, which on the good days didn't seem like forever. But of course on the bad days five minutes seemed like forever, but that's a whole other chapter.

As I mentioned before, you have to figure out how much weight you want to lose, and the best way to do this is to use the Body Mass Index (BMI) formula. You'll find this information at the beginning of Chapter 3. Once you've done this, next figure out how much time you want to take doing it, keeping in mind that a half to one kilo a week is the *most* you should lose in any given week.

One effective thing to do is to aim to have certain amounts of weight lost in time for particular events. Perhaps plan for your birthday or a friend's wedding. Having minor goals to work towards helps you focus your habits. Buy a dress that almost fits; keep trying it on; hang it somewhere you see it all the time. The closer you get, the more motivated you will be to reach that goal. But remember – be realistic. Don't give yourself three weeks to lose 10 kilos. No matter how many women say Princess Mary did it, it just isn't true!

Now that you've set your goals I want you to throw away any expectations you have and just get on with changing your life. It sounds like a contradiction, right? Well, it is. You *should* be goal-driven but you also have to accept things will happen that you have no control over. I broke my leg ten days into my 'diet'. I hadn't planned for that one, but I just got on with it any way I could, and still managed to keep losing weight.

There will be weeks when you don't lose weight. There will be weeks when you may actually put on weight. If you are exercising and working out there *will* be a time when the scales won't register a change but at these times you should ask yourself, 'what is my goal?' If it's health and fitness, and if you keep making healthy choices, and you keep your body moving, then no matter what the scales say you *are* achieving your goal.

7. Get focused — create your anchors

Anchors are catch phrases that support you in your journey. They are uplifting sayings, classic quotes and goals written down and pinned up where you will read them regularly. I find these to be extremely helpful. (Note: 'Chocolate bars are better than men' is not the kind of quote I am talking about.) I also repeat them out loud as often as I can just to reinforce the message. My favourite places are the toilet door, mirror, fridge door and kitchen cupboards. They're constant reminders that what you are doing is for the greater good. For example, before you open the fridge to grab your child's Caramello Koala you will see the sign 'What will look better on your hips? What you are about to eat or the sexy new jeans you'll fit into soon? Eat a piece of fruit instead!' On the fridge I had a Stop sign with the words 'Think about it. Do you really need this? Are you hungry or thirsty? Have some water instead'.

Near the front door I had: 'I am in control. I deserve a healthy body. I make healthy choices'. In the lounge room I had: 'Have you done your sit ups?' And beside the bed I had: 'I love myself, I honour my body. I deserve to be healthy and happy. Beer and battered savs are not God's gift to me'.

Change your anchors every couple of weeks to help you stay focused or when it's time to reassess your goals. My last boyfriend would go around and change them to things like 'It's OK, you found a man, you can get fat now' but that just motivated me to constantly rewrite them, which helped me refine and focus what it was I wanted and needed to do. He also wrote 'Making love is great exercise' . . . I left that one in place — a girl's gotta have some fun, and it is a great way to burn calories!

The idea behind the anchors is that you need constant reminders about what you are trying to achieve. Be your own personal trainer and motivator — that way you can save the money and spend it on sexy lingerie that doesn't have to double as a dust cover for a semi trailer!

8. Get moving. Go on, just do it.

Now all you need to do is get moving. I'm talking about exercise. Take baby steps. You can't do it overnight, and you can't do it all at once. For example, don't join a gym and do fifty classes in the first week. You'll either end up with a broken back or you'll be so exhausted you'll wind up disheartened and not prepared to go on. Remember, start slowly and realistically. You are on a very steep learning curve and all you can do is your best at each given time. When you make mistakes just keep going. Never give up on yourself. You can do it, I know you can. Now get off your fat bum and go for a walk.

Get started

- Do the pledge – every day.
- Get your health checked.
- Throw out all junk food.
- Drink some water.
- Go for a walk.
- Create a safe work and home environment.
- Take your 'before' photo (you will come to love it).
- Find a counsellor if you think you might need one. Find one anyway.
- Find a friend you can confide in and lean on.
- Go for a walk.
- Create your anchors – stick them everywhere.
- Start your food diary.
- Go for a walk. Right now. I mean it.

Quick Quiz

1. The best way to lose weight is:
   a) Not eat.
   b) Exercise for three hours a day and never eat anything you like.
   c) To watch your input versus your output. Have a little of every-
      thing and just keep going, no matter what happens.

2. Diets:
   a) Work well, but afterwards you always put the weight back on.
   b) Are too hard to stick to. You do them for two weeks but then get
      bored and crash and burn, ending up even bigger than you
      were before.
   c) Don't work. Only healthy eating and exercise works.

3. Low fat food:
   a) Is boring, and should only be fed to rabbits.
   b) Is tasteless.
   c) Can be anything you want it to be. It just takes a little extra effort.

Mostly a: Oh dear. We have an awful lot of work to do, haven't we? But
read on, there is hope for you yet.

Mostly b: Ah yes, you are like me. You have dieted yourself to a bigger
body. The sooner you stop 'dieting' the sooner you will have the body
and lifestyle you want.

Mostly c: At last! Someone who knows what I am talking about. But I'm
not sure what you are doing here. Maybe you have a fat friend who
should read this book.

3

The Basics, Part One

How much weight to lose, and what, how, and when to eat

'Any food eaten alone, or with the lights off, has zero calories.'
Fat Ajay

'Food is fuel and manicures are far better for me than Pluto Pups.'
Healthy Ajay

How big is your bum?

They say the truth hurts. Well, better get the Band Aids because this is that moment. Before you learn to eat well and move more you need to work out just how much weight, or fat, you are going to lose. I was so busy running around (or more truthfully, puffing around) calling myself a goddess that I had no idea that I was actually clinically and morbidly obese. Embarrassingly, I was too fat for the fat test at the gym – the calipers wouldn't fit around my gut. They couldn't even do the blood pressure test because my arm was too big for the stretchy elastic arm band. Hmm . . . that's why those Japanese whaling boats turned up every time I went for a swim!

When Crusher worked out how much weight I needed to lose I nearly died. She told me it was *at least* 40 kilos. Not possible, I thought. But it is possible, and it will seem a lot more achievable to you if you just break it down into smaller chunks. These days I advise my own clients to focus on just 5 kilos at a time. At the *most* you can healthily and realistically lose a kilo per week, but not any more than that – except in the first week when the weight just seems to drop off you (you can lose up to three kilos in those first seven days).

Swallow your pride and find out just how much you should lose, using the Body Mass Index formula, following. Then think about how much you will gain by getting healthy and taking control of your life.

Find out your Body Mass Index (BMI)

Your body mass index is a rough measure of your body fatness. The higher your BMI is, the more you risk developing high blood pressure, heart disease and diabetes. To de-jargonise it, your BMI works out just how much space you take up in relation to your height. If you are as wide as you are tall, then you may have a little bit of work to do.

The BMI formula can help you to work out roughly how much weight you should lose. Remember, though, your weight is an individual thing and just because a chart says you should be a certain weight does not mean you have to be exactly that. As long as you are fit and healthy it doesn't matter if you fall just outside the guidelines, but of course, if you can and want to get to the recommended weight, that's great, too.

I lift very heavy weights and carry a lot of muscle on my body so even though I fall between a size 10 and 12 (a shape I am happy with) the BMI formula still has me as being classed as 'overweight'. Now, I could diet my way down to the recommended weight for my height, but I prefer to be fit, healthy, strong, curvy and still have a few creature comforts like the occasional champagne and night out eating whatever I want. See? I told you about having your cake and eating it, too.

Your shape and size is a life choice – as long as you are *healthy*. And yes, I can hear someone saying it's their life choice to be a size 26, but by being that size they are not making a good life choice because chances are high that their quality of life will be compromised by heart disease and/or diabetes.

Working out your BMI is a simple equation:

$$BMI = \frac{Weight\ (kg)}{Height\ (m)^2}$$

For example, a 170 cm tall person is 75 kg. Their BMI = $\frac{75}{1.7 \times 1.7}$, which is $\frac{75}{2.89} = 25.9515571$

When that figure is rounded off to 26 it gets correlated to the height-to-weight classifications below, with recommendations of low, moderate, high and very high risk factors of how weight affects your health.

> 19 or under: Underweight
> 20–25: Healthy weight (low risk)
> 25–35: Overweight (moderate risk)
> 35–40: Obese (high risk)
> Over 40: Morbid obesity (very high risk)

As you can see our example is classified on the borderline between 'healthy' and 'overweight'. This person could probably afford to lose a little bit of weight, but then again, if they are muscly they are probably fine. This is when it comes down to personal choice and being sensible about how much weight to lose.

Now, if that person weighs 95 kilos we can do the same equation and see the results:

170 cm-tall person weighs 95 kg. Their BMI = $\frac{95}{1.7 \times 1.7}$, which is $\frac{95}{2.89}$ = 32.8719723

When that figure is rounded off to 33 you can see our candidate is now classed at the top end of 'overweight' and very close to becoming obese. The BMI calculation is a quick way to give yourself a bit of a reality check, and if you fall into the last two categories there is no time to lose — you have to start moving now! There are *no* excuses.

In order to work out roughly how much you need or want to lose, first of all aim for the higher end of your projected BMI. Then I want you to add 5 kilos. Say, for instance, that you are 160 cm tall. Your 'healthy weight' BMI would have you somewhere between 52 and 62 kilos. If you have over 20 kilos to lose then I want your long-term goal to be 67 kilos. Of course, if you are already 67 kilos then aim for 62 and just do it. But for those with a long way to go you need to be realistic. You may get to 67 and still want to lose those extra kilos, which is great. But you may also get to 67 and absolutely love the body you have.

Now, if you truly are a lazy girl and don't want to (or couldn't be bothered) working out your BMI, type 'BMI calculator' into Google and you'll be directed to many sites that can do it for you in three seconds flat.

Above all else, when it comes to calculating your BMI, don't let it trick you into thinking that you are not good enough. I have a friend who looks like Brad Pitt (yes, it is a pity about the 'friend' bit. Sigh). He is buffed. Really buffed. Imagine the bedroom scene in *Troy* and you are on the right track. Now his BMI reading has him as obese. Let me tell you right now, this man is *not* obese. I haven't looked under his toga but there doesn't seem to be anything that shouldn't be there, or be the size it is. (Well . . . apart from *one* thing!) But he *is* muscly and as I have said before, muscle is denser, or heavier than fat. Therefore the BMI is completely irrelevant to him. He couldn't care less about the BMI.

Similarly, I know a personal trainer who has a body to die for. She is fit, healthy, curvy, muscly and strong. She works out like a demon, runs high energy fitness classes four times a day, six times a week and she looks great. She recently did the BMI test which told her she was obese, and now she's dissatisfied with her body. Now she wants to lose a lot of weight, and fast. The most sensible road ahead for her would be to focus on losing just 5 kilos, which will leave her body more defined and streamlined without the negative self or body image. *Then* she can decide whether to lose more.

You need to know that the BMI calculation is only a rough guide. Do not live or die by it, or should I say live or diet by it. The goal is health and fitness, not a specific weight or size. Now, I know that you have just worked out your BMI and calculated just how much you need to lose. Your head is probably spinning, you have fallen into a pit of despair, the whole way ahead seems impossible and you can't see the light at the end of the tunnel.

Do not give up. The only way out is through. *Don't* focus on the bigger picture. Do what I tell everyone in the Healthy Body Club to do: focus on 5 kilos at a time. You can lose 5 kilos in five weeks. Mark it in your diary for five weeks from now. See yourself there. Remember, the trick is to break your weight loss into smaller, achievable amounts. If you want to do it slowly, do 5 kilos in eight weeks. Just make sure you focus and reward yourself every little step along the way.

The wonderful thing is that in the first week you can

expect to lose up to 3 kilos, but it *will* drop down after that. I've mentioned this before, but health professionals recommend a *maximum* weight loss of 1 kilo per week. If you consistently lose any more than that it is not healthy, or sustainable. So many women check in and are disappointed that they have 'only' lost a kilo or half a kilo. But 1 kilo is three tubs of margarine! Have a look at, and feel how heavy, half a kilo of potatoes is and you will see your weight loss very differently.

Remember, the faster you do it the faster it will come racing back to your thighs. Doing it slowly and sensibly is more permanent. I lost 45 kilos in one year. That is what I mean by 'slowly', and it isn't such a snail's pace when you look at the big picture, is it? Eight dress sizes in one year. That allowed for a few treats, a few weekends away, weight put on when I was building muscle and any attempts at sabotage. Twelve months: that's all it takes to go from a size 26 to a size 12. It's a whole new life, a different way to live, think, feel and be.

Changing how you eat

Next, now that you've broken up with chocolate, thrown out the Tim Tams (do it) and taken the pledge (do it), it's time to start eating. Yes, I am very serious.

I recently went out to dinner and there was an obese woman sitting next to me. While we were lining up for the buffet one of her friends commented that she eats like a sparrow. I was immediately suspicious. I imagined a huge cartoon sparrow as big as Hagrid in *Harry Potter*. I watched what she put on her plate. She stacked it with roast beef, baked potatoes, pasta and three bread rolls. That was some sparrow! When we started talking she admitted it was her one and only meal of the day. I used to be guilty of that. I would only have one meal – but it could feed a small nation.

Almost every person I consult with at The Healthy Body Club doesn't eat breakfast, often skips meals, never eats snacks and eats more at the tail end of the day than the start. When I was obese I'd be lucky to eat before midday, then I'd make up for lost time and eat for three.

The problem with going for long periods of time without food is that your body goes into starvation mode. As soon as you put food in your mouth it stores it as fat straight away because it doesn't know how long it will be before your next meal. Your metabolism slows down, and not only doesn't burn any of the fat on your body, but also stores everything you eat as fat as well. It gets the message that there is a famine and that it needs to store food (as fat) because there may not be another meal for a long time. You need to get your metabolism burning again and the easiest way to do that is to *eat* and *eat regularly*.

Eat!

You need to create a new healthy eating plan which means having breakfast, snack, lunch, snack, dinner, and snack, the last being optional depending on when you are going to bed. I know this seems like a lot, and I know you don't believe me, but I didn't believe Crusher either. When she looked over my food diary she declared that I had to eat more, and more often. I, like every other woman in the world, believed that you had to eat less to lose weight. I'd subscribed to the Starve Yourself To Get Thin Club, which really only makes you sick, or eventually fatter. It wasn't until I started eating regular meals that I actually started to lose weight. So eat, dammit!

The first thing I set my Clubbers (Healthy Body Club members) is what I call The Breakfast Challenge. Get up and eat breakfast as soon as you can. You need to train your body to become a lean, mean, fat-burning machine. If you eat every three to four hours your body learns that is it being fed regularly. Then, when you start moving, it knows it can burn that excess fat from your body.

I don't mean roll out of bed and into a bowl of Cornflakes but you need to eat within half an hour of waking, and, of course, your breakfast choice needs to be healthy and low fat. I know you are not hungry in the morning and would rather slam your left breast in a car door than eat but you have to trust me on this. The reason you are not hungry is because you have trained your body not to eat. Your metabolism has come to a standstill and has probably stored your last meal from the night before as fat, knowing it won't eat till whenever it is you take your first bite of food.

Most of the women I consult with have got into the habit of not eating till mid-morning, but after a week of the breakfast challenge they are waking up starving and want to eat the first thing they lay their eyes on – even if it is their first born. Those who take the breakfast challenge (and change nothing else) still manage to lose roughly 2–3 kilos in the first week. As soon as you eat, your metabolism starts working and burning fat. Your hunger will increase and in the first few weeks you should start seeing a dramatic change in your weight.

The other common thing most people do is skip their snacks, once again using the excuse that they are not hungry. But the more often you eat, the hungrier you will get. Again, your snacks have to be healthy, low fat choices and not a bucket of KFC, but if you keep eating regularly your body will keep burning fat. Don't let your body run out of fuel. As soon as you do your metabolism will shut down and go back to storing food as fat.

You have to remind your body to be hungry and sometimes you just have to force yourself to eat at your designated meal times. If you do this you *will* lose weight.

How much to eat

'All You Can Eat meal deals are out. Up-sizing is out. Eating for three is out.' Even though I knew I had to cut down my calories that was pretty much the sum total of my knowledge on how to lose weight healthily. I used to read diet books and fall asleep at page three. But losing weight isn't that hard. It's simply Input versus Output.

I'm not going to prattle on with all the jargon you read in diet books. Diets don't work. The bottom line is, if you cut down your calorie and fat intakes and get moving, you *will* lose your big bum.

Aim at consuming around 1200–1400 calories a day. Within that you should have between 40 and 60 grams of fat per day. That's it – all the information you need to take your life back. Well, it's not really that simple; if it was there wouldn't be a fat person in the world. The key is to work out the simple stuff (your intake) and then you can work on the other stuff (why you want to consume three times your intake in just one meal).

The human body will consume around 2200 calories per day (this is based on an 18–35 year-old woman weighing approximately 75 kg). If you reduce your calorie intake to 1400 calories per day you are already using your excess body weight to find those extra calories you need to get through the day. You have started losing weight. Once you add exercise to

Calories for weight loss

Women	(no exercise)	1000–1200
	(exercising)	1200–1400
Men	(no exercise)	1200–1500
	(exercising)	1500–1800

the mix you are heading towards your goal of making significant and permanent life changes to your body.

Now, if you are anything like I was you need to find out just what you can and can't eat. Low fat is excellent. Low sugar is great. Low calorie choices are better than high calorie, but I can hear you ask, 'How do I know what's what?'

You are about to become the Eliza Doolittle of calories and fat. You need to educate yourself about everything you put in your mouth. Very soon you will know what food is 'good' and 'bad', you will know roughly how many calories and how much fat you are consuming on a daily basis and you will know when to treat yourself and when to go easy. You will know all of this without having to read a label, check a book or weigh and measure your food. I promise.

You don't need to obsess. I never counted up exactly how many calories I consumed. There were no scenes in restaurants where I pulled out my calculator, prodded the food with a pen and weighed it with my scales. I did a rough estimate. And after a while I knew how many calories a piece of pizza contained and it didn't seem that attractive. Knowing what you are eating in terms of calories and fat makes it easier to make healthy choices.

Buy yourself a calorie counter. This is a little pocket-sized book that lists the calorie and fat contents of most foods, including take-aways. Have a read of the fast food section and you will think twice about ever stepping inside one of those places again. When you discover you can have a healthy dinner for 14 grams of fat versus one Krispy Kreme donut for 20 grams you start to see food in a whole new light, or should I say lite. If you eat three donuts you have blown your whole day's fat intake. Also, while you've got your wallet out, buy some slimming magazines: they have great handy hints, lots of excellent meal plans, recipes and great suggestions of low fat alternatives for the foods you love to eat. Also, pick up every *Women's Weekly* low fat cookbook you can find. They have at least six in their range and they are all excellent.

It's amazing how many people think they are eating healthily but are actually consuming two or three times their daily intake of fat. A friend of mine was eating soy chips because she thought that anything with soy was good for you. Unfortunately they were deep-fried and one packet contained 60 grams of fat. She was having three packets of these a day and couldn't understand why she was putting on weight despite exercising and 'watching what she ate'.

Someone else was eating fifteen pieces of chocolate every night and having scones for breakfast. Scones are made with butter and flour; and chocolate is the enemy – and the truth is you are going to have to break up with it. You can still see it as a friend but there will be no more late night fumbling in the bed or in front of the TV.

Warning! Depressing piece of information following: a Mars Bar has 14 grams of fat, which is roughly what your main meal of the day should be. Now don't get me wrong – you can have a Mars Bar occasionally. But for now, you'll be a lot better off without them.

As you can see, once you start getting your head around

the amounts of fat and calories you're eating, it's easy to feel motivated to make the right choices that will really kick your weight loss into action. Also, knowing what you're eating means that you are being honest with yourself and taking responsibility. Ignorance is for those who don't want to achieve their goals.

Plan to eat

Before you do your weekly shopping, look through your low fat recipe books. If you haven't got any, put them on your shopping list, or have a quick flick through the recipes or the four week eating plan I've included at the back of the book. Decide which great meals you are going to cook, and have fun with it. Try not to feel daunted by it – most low fat recipes are very easy and fast to make and the majority are delicious and yummy enough for your partner and/or kids to eat as well. Make the nights you're cooking special by setting up a romantic, candle-lit table for you and your partner and one (only one) glass of wine. Praise your kids for eating healthy food that will make them grow up big and strong like Super-man, or with those amazing bosoms Wonderwoman has (just kidding). It doesn't have to be a chore; you're changing your life for the better, so make it fun and worthwhile.

Once you've decided what you're going to cook, write up a menu plan for all your meals for the week, including your snacks and a few Lean Cuisines just while you get the hang of things. Your menu plan gives you something to look forward to, because you know what you'll be eating, and it staves off any opportunities for you to come off the wagon. Write down your shopping list, including lots of fruit and low fat yoghurt for your snacks.

Also, consult your calorie counter before you go shopping, or even at the supermarket. It's particularly good when you're deciding what snacks to buy. Check out the best options, like which yoghurt has the lowest calories and fat; decide exactly what it is you are going to consume. Doing this will help you make better choices all round. I leave my calorie counter on my coffee table and flick through it whenever I'm bored. It helps educate me about all the choices I have, including those when I'm out and about. Remember, this is a permanent change you are making to your eating habits, and you are simply teaching yourself about what healthy food is. One day soon you will know what healthy food is very well, and won't have to consult so much with cookbooks or the counter.

There is hope

The great thing is that, these days, you can get most foods in a fat free or low fat version. I even found low fat hot dogs (less than 2 grams of fat!) and low fat sour cream (Paul's Diet Sour Cream – 1 tablespoon has only 0.6 grams of fat). If you want something desperately enough you will find a healthy way to do it. Losing weight and getting fit is not about denying yourself everything or never having the food you like. It's not about enduring a certain amount of time eating only one thing then reverting back to your bad old ways. It's about finding healthy ways to eat the food you love and knowing when, and when not to, lash out. Everything in moderation is OK. Nothing is totally banned.

This is a way of life, not a way to a life.

The changes you are making in your life are permanent so you will be better off spending a bit of time finding a healthy alternative than going without until you crash and burn, have too much then give up on yourself. That is the diet yo-yo cycle. Get off it and start learning to live your life healthily.

Control your fat intake

Controlling your fat intake is the best thing you can do to lose weight. Excess fat is stored as fat. It's as simple as that. Let me say it again: *Fat is stored as fat.* You don't want to have to keep working it off for the rest of your life – just lose it and then don't put any more on. You can do this by learning to eat healthy alternatives and sticking to your designated daily fat intake. That's it. The 'secret' to weight loss.

Daily intake of fat

No, I'm not talking about how many times you have to look at yourself in the mirror, I'm talking about how much fat is in the food you eat. Some foods are high in fat, some have little to none. Eating a combination of foods allows you to have variety, sustenance, adequate nutrition and some foods simply because you like them.

For women, the daily intake of fat should be roughly 40–60 grams (maximum) per day. A rough break-down of fat consumed over a day should read something like this:

> **Breakfast:** 5–8 grams
> **Snack:** up to 5 grams
> **Lunch:** 10 grams
> **Snack:** up to 5 grams
> **Dinner:** 10–15 grams
> **Snack:** up to 5 grams

For men, fat intake can be slightly higher – 40–80 g per day.

This is a rough guide only. Once you know what you are eating you can chop and change and make choices throughout the day, which will depend on where you are and what you are doing. For example, a lunch higher in fat would mean a dinner lower in fat. Planning your fat intake this way means you can have a few of the things you love and never really go without. Constantly balance your meals so you still consume the same amount of fat every day.

I imagine my fat intake as my son's piggy bank (appropriate, don't you think?). Every time I eat something I add up how much I have put into the piggy bank. It only holds 60 'coins', so as the day goes by I have to be careful I don't overload it as the pig will break open from having too much in there. If you keep an eye on your calories and your fat content you can't really go wrong. After that, it's a matter of exercising, working on your habits, controlling your emotional eating and then you will have the body of your dreams. Just like that. Poof! God, I love the fat fairy.

What's that? You don't believe me? I promise you it *is* as simple as that. I dieted all of my adult life but it wasn't until I focused on one thing at a time and backed it up by eating healthily (with treats) and exercise that I lost eight dress sizes from my body. One year is all it took. Sixteen years of dieting versus one year of eating well. I am the living proof that you *can* change your life by taking it one day at a time, one meal at a time. And no, you're not allowed to say 'It was easy for her'. Everyone can do this – just give it a go.

Nutrition guides

Apart from having a calorie counter, what else can you do to find out how much fat is in your food? Read the nutrition guide on the packet. Most packaged food has one and it's a breakdown of the nutrition in it in percentages. The things you need to note are the energy values (calories/kJ), the fat (in grams) and how many serves are in the packet. Here's one for bread, below.

BREAD NUTRITION INFORMATION SERVES PER PACKAGE: 9		
Serving Size: 85 g (2 slices)	Average Quantity Per Serving	Average Quantity Per 100 g
Energy	815 kJ	974 kJ
Protein	8.6 g	10.3 g
Fat, Total	2.3 g	2.8 g
– Saturated	0.4 g	0.5 g
Carbohydrate	31.8 g	38.1 g
– Sugars	1.8 g	2.1 g
Dietary fibre	4.9 g	5.9 g
Sodium	313 mg	375 mg

Most nutritional panels have two columns, one explaining the nutrition breakdown per serve and the other the nutrition per 100 grams. For example, say you have two crumpets with light peanut butter for afternoon tea. You check the nutrition guides. One tablespoon (serve 20 g) of light peanut butter is 466 kJ (roughly 110 calories) and has 7.6 g of fat. Crumpets also have 335 kJ and 0.5 g of fat each. If you have two tablespoons of peanut butter on two crumpets you have consumed more than triple the fat, and four times the calorie allowance for just one snack. (If you're wondering how to convert kilojoules to calories, just divide by four and add a bit – that's how I do it, or see page 320.)

Alternatively when you read the guide for Marmite you find the same serve has 9 calories and only 0.4 grams of fat. Now which spread do you think you should choose? It's not the peanut butter. That becomes a treat – have it once a week instead of every day. *Having the knowledge gives you the power.* It takes thirty seconds to read what you are about to eat and about five years to work those extras calories off – but if you stop the excess going in, you'll have a chance to work the excess off, and keep it off.

Don't be tricked into eating more than you should

Be aware that there can be numerous serves per package – for instance, most regular tubs of yoghurt actually contain two serves. Also, beware that something proclaiming to have only 9 grams of fat may actually have that per 100 grams – if the serving size is 300 grams in total you could be consuming a total of 27 grams of fat for dinner or lunch.

Also, don't get sucked into the '50% less fat than regular variation' trap. This doesn't mean it is necessarily low in fat; it could still contain 30% fat. For example, one popular sauce-in-a-jar range still contains up to 28% fat. Once you add the chicken and cheese you have blown two days' calories in one single meal! It doesn't mean you have to go without, but it might mean that you significantly reduce your portion and add salad to bulk up your meal.

It's also important to keep an eye on *all* low fat products. Certain brands proclaim to be 'diet' but they may not be the *lowest* in fat. When buying light margarine check all the labels and you'll be surprised which ones are actually the lowest in fat. For example, a popular brand of diet spread is 5.5 grams of fat per teaspoon, whereas Western Star Lite Butter is only 2 grams of fat for the same amount. Don't be told what to buy by manufacturers – work it out yourself.

Also 'lite' food does not necessarily mean light in fat. 'Lite' olive oil means light in colour. 'Lite' can mean light in salt. The term 'light and crispy' is used with a lot of frozen fish meals but not all of them refer to the fat content; some mean light and crispy in texture. These are clever marketing techniques but the nutrition guide will tell all, generally.

A good balance

It's important to find out what is best for you and then make an educated choice from what's available. Pre-packaged, delivered-to-your-door diets are not permanent weight loss solutions. What do you do when you've lost the weight? What do you do when you have a family? What do you do when you have a dinner party? It's so much easier to learn low fat recipes and make permanent life choices so that being healthy is just a part of living normally. That's all I ever wanted to be – normal. I'm not sure I will ever achieve that, but I do eat 'normally' now . . . most of the time.

It's also worth having a look at the sugar content of the food you eat, too, although I would rather you eat food higher in sugar than higher in fat. Low on both counts would be perfect, but who are we kidding here? Lettuce leaves and carrot sticks are for rabbits. I can't get by without my red licorice and jelly snakes. What you need to find is a balance of healthy choices, allowable treats and luxury foods backed up with an exercise plan. *That* is the recipe for a healthy, happy life. How much grief is wrapped up in so-called comfort food? How many times have you hated yourself for what you have just eaten? Food should be fuel first of all, then used as a comfort only occasionally. I never thought I would get to the point where 90 per cent of my meals contained no emotional baggage. It makes me feel 10 kilos lighter just not having to stress over what's going into my body. If you persevere, food will no longer be your entire world – it will be what you need to get through the day, and occasionally the luxury that it has the capacity to be.

What, when and how to eat

Breakfast
As I have mentioned, this is the most important meal of the day and is *not* negotiable.

Every day you should eat within half an hour of waking up. Start by having something small like low-fat yoghurt or a banana. In a few days you will wake up feeling very hungry. When this happens you can move up to a small bowl of high fibre cereal and fruit, or a low fat smoothie and toast. *Do not miss this meal.*

Snack (mid-morning)
Remember, having snacks will keep your metabolism burning. Keep it fuelled to keep it firing.

Don't be sucked into eating tempting treats that are high in calories but not very filling. Trade your snacks up and make better choices by consuming the same amount of calories for a bigger serving of food. Two pieces of fruit and some low fat yoghurt will equal the same amount of calories but less fat than one popular brand of muffin bar, which is 9 grams of fat.

Lunch
This is an important meal. You need enough fuel to get you through the rest of the day and to avoid multiple afternoon snacking sessions.

Low-fat sandwiches, soup or pasta are great choices at this time of day. Fill your sandwiches up with lots of salad and avoid fatty sandwich meats. Salad makes you feel full. If you are still hungry after eating a sandwich then have a cup of low-fat or vegetable soup or a piece of fruit.

Snack (afternoon)
Again, this meal is important because it will give you enough fuel to make it through to dinner, but more importantly it will stop you from making bad choices at dinner. When we are 'starving' it is harder to make rational choices so we go for less healthy foods, prefer to comfort eat, and often eat twice as much as we should. If you have a sufficiently healthy snack in the afternoon, getting to and through dinner time without a blow-out should not be a problem.

Again, fruit or low-fat yoghurt is best at this time of the day. If you get really hungry again and it is still two hours till dinner then have a second afternoon snack like a cup of soup or low-fat hot chocolate drink, or even another piece of fruit. Make sure that if you do double snack, it is low in sugar and fat.

Dinner
Go easy. Dinner shouldn't be your biggest meal of the day as you are just going to lie in bed and there isn't much opportunity for burning off calories (that is, unless you have a night of mattress aerobics planned!). Eat well, but don't overeat.

Before I started on my weight loss kick I was the takeaway queen. This changed pretty quickly! You need to learn how to cook quick and easy, healthy, low fat meals. Believe it or not it's not as hard as you think. I set myself small goals – in the first few weeks I relied heavily on Lean Cuisines with added salad or steamed vegetables. I knew I couldn't live like that forever so I taught myself two new low fat meals per week. I bought about ten low fat recipe books, I looked on the internet and in slimming magazines for recipes, and I picked up recipe sheets from the supermarket. These days I can cook from normal cookbooks and convert the recipe to low fat without too much trouble.

Snack

This after dinner snack is purely optional. It can be dessert if you want. It can also bridge the gap between dinner and breakfast, particularly if you are having a late night. However, you should not snack two hours or less before bedtime because all you are going to do is lie in bed and sleep.

If you are getting hungry just before you go to bed, you need to readjust when you eat. For example, say you are getting to bed at midnight. Your dinner was at seven. If you eat again at eleven, you are going to bed with food that just lies around in your tummy, not being metabolised. Instead, think about when you are going to get to bed. If you know it is midnight then have a healthy snack at 9 pm therefore curbing your before-bed hunger. These snacks can't be sugar or chocolate though – it is too late in the day to have this kind of food – your body has no chance to burn it off. Fruit or yoghurt is best. If you find yourself constantly wanting food at this time then get a low fat hot chocolate drink that mixes up with water. (Jarrah is my personal favourite.) It will comfort you through this period and become your new late night habit.

Meal ideas

For those with no idea about what to eat, here are some suggestions for three days. As you can see, I've included the calorie and fat breakdowns for each meal and the totals for each day, so you can see what these foods roughly count up to in terms of daily calorie and fat expenditures. If you're after some more ideas, or want a more structured plan, have a look at the four-week eating plan at the back of the book. In all cases, always choose low fat or skim dairy, lean protein

Day 1

Breakfast	Calories	Fat (g)
Low fat strawberry smoothie, 1 slice of toast Vegemite (no margarine or butter)	300	7
Snack		
Low fat yoghurt, small banana	140	0.2
Lunch		
Subway Chicken Roll (Under 6'')	140	2
Snack		
10 grapes, 8 whole raw almonds	120	4
Dinner		
Lean Cuisine plus salad with low fat dressing or vegetables, including one oven-baked potato	560	13
Snack		
Weight Watchers ice cream (small cup)	130	0.2
Total	1390	26.4

Day 2

Breakfast	Calories	Fat (g)
Poached egg on 1 slice of toast, 1 small banana	160	6
Snack		
Half a punnet of strawberries, with Nestle Diet Chocolate Mousse	80	1.5
Lunch		
Vegetable soup, 1 slice of toast, 1 apple	310	5
Snack		
Handful of baked pretzels, 1 kiwifruit	190	1
Dinner		
Grilled fillet of fish, salad with low fat dressing	250	3
Snack		
Diet jelly	30	0
Total	1020	16.5

Day 3		
Breakfast	Calories	Fat (g)
Small bowl high fibre cereal, with low fat milk,		
yoghurt, fresh fruit	160	2
Snack		
Small apple and 2 red licorice strips	180	0.5
Lunch		
Small serve of pasta with tomato-based sauce	260	8
Snack		
3 sardines in springwater on 3 regular sized		
Vitaweets	175	6.5
Dinner		
Grilled chicken breast, steamed veggies,		
1/3 cup of steamed rice	350	10
Snack		
Weight watchers ice cream	130	0.2
Total	**1255**	**27.2**

(cut the fat off meat, or choose ultra trim cuts), lots of fruit and veggies, and use no, or very little, oil or margarine.

As you embark on your healthy eating plan, keep an eye on your daily calorie and fat totals and they will let you know when and how much to treat yourself. For example, if you've already had 45 grams of fat during the day and have yet to eat dinner, that Mars Bar of 14 grams of fat doesn't look as good or as satisfying, compared to a Lean Cuisine (12 grams of fat) and veggies and salad for dinner. However, if you've only had 25 grams of fat during the day, that Mars Bar may look a little more reasonable if you make sure you stick to the Lean Cuisine for dinner. Remember, though, a piece of fruit is *always* better than a Mars Bar!

Oh, and don't run out of food. Ever. If there is no food in the house, you will end up bingeing and splurging. Buy fresh fruit and veggies every couple of days, and have plenty of staples on hand (e.g. baked beans, cans of tuna, tins of tomatoes, bread). It's much easier to just go to the cupboard and eat whatever is on hand than fantasising about what you want and then rushing out to buy it. *Always be prepared*.

Food serves

Remember the good old healthy food pyramid we have known for most of our lives? It's a great guide to how much fruit, veggies, meat, fat and dairy you should eat through the day, ensuring you get the best possible nutrition and health benefits from the food you eat. I bet you've seen that picture a million times and I bet you still don't know how many serves of fruit you are supposed to have every day. And even if you do know, I bet you don't live by it.

The truth is, you do need to implement the information from the pyramid into your life. This knowledge is the foundation for all the other work you will do. Every fat chick knows she should eat more fruit and veggies, and less fat. That's no big secret. So why don't we do it? Because we couldn't be bothered being a healthy person. We want to be the same old lazy girl *and* be thin, happy, healthy and content. This is what I mean about having a reality check. You need to *become* a healthy person and the only way you can do that is to start feeding yourself good food, get moving and retrain your brain.

If you try your very best to eat like a healthy person, you will become one. Just bluff it until you become it; that's what I did. And I know you might not like veggies (yet) – been there, done that! I tackled one vegetable at a time. I tried them in soups, then in casseroles and healthy curries, sandwiches, salads and then in all the other food I had never tried. I *thought* I didn't like vegetables but that wasn't true. I just didn't like vegetables the way my mother had served them.

I have since learned to cook them myself and now love a lot of them. I am still no devotee of pumpkin or brussel sprouts but there is more to life than those two veggies.

The same goes for fruit. Once you get into the habit of eating the right kind of food you feel much more energised. Just see it as a habit you have to make. Once it's a habit, you'll love what it does for you. I always say to Kai, 'It's a new thing. You might like it.' Sometimes he does like it and sometimes he spits it out quicker than John Wayne spat out chewing tobacco, but at least he tries it. You should too. It's a new thing. You might like it.

The basics

According to the food pyramid, every day you should have:

- 3 serves of **lean** protein (e.g. beef, lamb, pork and veal, fish, chicken, turkey, tofu, legumes, etc)
- 2 serves of **low fat** dairy products (e.g. cheese, milk, yoghurt, etc)
- 2–3 serves of carbohydrates, like bread, grains, cereals, etc
- 2–3 serves of fruit
- 4 serves of vegetables
- 1 serve of (good) fat (and I don't mean a Quarter Pounder and fries). These fats can be found in olive oil, nuts, seeds, fish, avocado, etc.

Food diary

The food diary really is a must do (see page 280 for yours). And no, I am *not* talking about all the sordid dreams you have of covering Keanu in chocolate body paint, or those sexy late night imaginings of Johnny Depp and a bucket of whipped cream, strawberries and red licorice whips. I'm talking about writing down every little thing you eat and drink.

There's nothing like having a good, hard, honest look at what and how much you eat during the day. Like learning how much fat is in what you eat, finding out how, when and how much you eat can teach you so much about yourself. It wasn't until I started writing things down that I realised that I would go for five or six hours without eating – and then, starving, I would eat twice as much as I should have. Because I hadn't eaten for so long my body didn't know when the next meal was going to be and simply turned everything I ate into fat.

Once I focused on writing everything down the first thing it did was remind me to eat, and more importantly, eat at the right times. It made me think ahead, too, about what I was going to eat through the day. It also helped me work out when I was going to get hungry and taught me to prepare for those times.

Knowing I was recording everything I was more likely to (attempt to) make healthy choices, and when I crumbled I could have a good look at what had gone wrong. Over the weeks I could see trends in my eating that would help me refocus and refine what I was doing.

For example, the most common thing for everyone is to overeat on the weekends. Knowing that would happen, I would plan to have the right kind of food on hand and make an extra special effort to remain focused and write down what I ate. If you don't write it down those calories and fat units can add up without you ever really knowing just how much you have consumed.

The great thing about your food diary is you can adjust what you eat to compensate for things you have already eaten in a day, a few days, or over a whole week. For example, be mindful of your fat and calorie 'allowance' over the day. If you get close to using your entire allowance by lunch-time then you'll need to make really healthy choices for the next two meals to keep you within your fat and calorie ranges. For example, your next snack can be fruit, and dinner can be chunky vegetable soup or a big salad – all these choices have low calories and, even better, no fat.

If certain foods keep cropping up in your food diary and they are sabotaging your weight loss, then focus on finding a remedy. Don't get depressed that you keep craving, and then eating, hot chips. Find a solution. Make fat free wedges and have them as your weekly reward.

When you have kept a diary for six weeks or so, have a look over the weeks and see how your eating changes when you are premenstrual, and then menstrual. Mark it on your diary a few days before you are due and make sure you are prepared for any hormonal blow-outs.

Most importantly, though, tally up your fat and calorie intakes at the end of each day and constantly analyse and refine the choices you are making – if you stay within your allowances, you *will* lose weight; there are no two ways about it. It's also good to see how you are going emotionally. Notice how you feel about yourself having had a good healthy day versus having a bad blow-out day. This knowledge can be the key to unlocking your mind, and subsequently your body.

Diary examples

Following are two examples of two very different food diaries. These are typical first weeks: both people want to lose weight, have made drastic changes to their eating habits, and thought they were making healthy choices. They're great to look at because you can see where each made a good choice, or a not-so-good choice. My comments are in bold.

Diary One

Tuesday

B: 2 date scones, butter, coffee. *Scones are full of butter; also use lite butter, or none at all.*
S: Rockmelon. *Add yoghurt.*
L: Small chicken pasta, broccoli, and pumpkin. *Excellent lunch.*
S: K-Time bar. *Plus fruit/yoghurt.*
D: 3 crumbed fish (oven-roasted), wedges (large), tartar sauce, chilli sauce. *Check the fat content. You may have had 40 g fat in one meal.*
S: 8 chocolate squares, 15 Pringles, 1 mini Kit-Kat. *Oops!*
Exercise: –

Wednesday

B: 2 date scones, butter, coffee. *Again, scones are full of butter; use lite butter or margarine, or none at all.*
S: Hot chocolate (skim milk). *Food needed here.*
L: Boiled rice, chilli chicken. *Check fat content.*
S: *Eat!*
D: 3 fish (oven-roasted), 5 wedges, tartar sauce, sweet chilli sauce. *Again, check fat content.*
S: 4 choc squares, 1 mini Mars Bar. *Oops!*
Exercise: Gym – cardio and weights.

Thursday

B: Banana smoothie (banana and skim milk). *Excellent breakfast!*
S: *Eat!*
L: 1 small and 1 medium burger. *Oops!*
S: *Eat!*
D: Pad Thai, large boiled rice. *Watch the takeaway. Pad Thai is high in fat. Next time try a veggie and chicken stir-fry.*
S: 8 chocolate squares. *Oops! Once a week maybe, not every day.*
Exercise: Gym – cardio and weights.

Friday

B: Yoghurt, Sultana Bran, lite milk, 2 x Burgen bread, butter, honey 1 tsp. *Excellent breakfast!*
S: Orange. *Plus yoghurt.*
L: Chicken Pad Thai. *Again, watch high fat takeaways.*
S: *Eat.*
D: Lean chicken tart, peas, corn. *Great dinner.*
S: 2 mini choc eggs, 1 mini Kit Kat. *No more chocky! Make it once a week only.*
Exercise: Walk (30 min).

Saturday

B: 2 date scones, butter, coffee. *Scones full of butter; use lite butter or margarine.*

S: Skim hot chocolate. *Great! But food needed, too.*

L: Boiled rice, Mongolian chicken. *Watch fat content.*

S: *Food needed here.*

D: Lean Cuisine. *You can add veggies.*

S: Crème caramel (diet). *Have a piece of fruit, too.*

Exercise: –

Sunday

B: Mushrooms, bacon, eggs, tomato, coffee. *Cut fat off bacon, poach eggs.*

S: *Eat.*

L: Sausage, bread roll, onions, chilli, BBQ sauce, wine (1). *Sausages are no good (roughly 20% fat); but 1 glass wine is fine.*

S: 1 cinnamon roll, skim cappuccino. *Fruit a better choice.*

D: Panang Chicken, large boiled rice. *Again, watch the high fat takeaways.*

S: 4 choc squares. *No, once a week.*

Monday

B: Yoghurt, Sultana Bran, lite milk, 2 x Burgen bread, butter, honey. *Excellent.*

S: Skim hot chocolate. *Have a piece of fruit, too.*

L: Small tomato pasta, broccoli, pumpkin. *Great lunch.*

S: K Twist. *Plus yoghurt or fruit.*

D: Rice pudding and banana. *How about a salad?*

S: 2 mini choc eggs. *No more chocky!*

Exercise: Gym – weights and cardio.

Sum-up of the week

This person did some great exercise but what's the point if there was so much extra fat consumed? They need to stop eating the chocolate, especially at night. Chocolate should be once a week only, or one square a day. They also need to eat more fruit, and all their day snacks. They need to choose stir-fries and avoid packaged food – even 'oven-roasted' things like wedges. This person will not have lost weight. They need to ask themselves if they really want to lose the weight, because you cannot consume that much fat and chocolate every day and expect to lose weight. The good thing is they can go over their food diary and circle all the foods they should cut out or down. They also need to find alternative ways to feel good or nurture themselves, instead of eating comfort food.

Diary Two

Tuesday

B: 1 K-Time bar. *How about cereal, fruit and yoghurt?*
S: Mandarin and box of sultanas. *Great!*
L: 1x 98% fat free lunch-time pasta, apple and mandarin.
D: 98% fat free noodles.
S: Grapes, 4 Snack Right biscuits.
Exercise: 150 sit-ups, personal training session, 15 minutes on the treadmill.

Wednesday

B: 1 K-Time bar. *Again, eat more please.*
S: Mandarin.
L: Big salad with avocado and tuna.
S: Apple, mandarin.
D: Low fat seafood pizza.
S: –
Exercise: –

Thursday

B: Apple, mandarin. *Need to eat more, like toast and yoghurt as well.*
S: Apple.
L: Lean Cuisine with tomato salad.
S: Mandarin.
D: 4 sushi rolls.
S: Frozen mango drink.
Comments: Had dinner in food court.
Exercise: 150 sit-ups.

Friday

B: Apple. *Plus more food!*
S: Mandarin.
L: 3 sushi rolls.
S: 2 sushi rolls.
D: Antipasto + bread, ½ grilled chicken breast with salsa.
S: 1 Lemon Ruski, 1 white wine.
Comments: Restaurant for dinner, and to a bar with friends later.
Exercise: 150 sit-ups.

Saturday

B: 2 slices of toast with Vegemite. *More food needed.*
S: Handful of grapes.
L: 2 grilled prawn skewers .*You could add a salad here.*
S: 10 pistachios.
D: Grilled barramundi and salad.
S: –
Comments: Happy, went to the fish markets for lunch and instead of the seafood platter, had the healthy option. Still yummy!
Exercise: 150 sit-ups.

Sunday

B: Bowl of low fat yoghurt with fruit. *Great choice!*
S: Apple.
L: 2 scrambled eggs on 2 slices toast.
S: 10 pistachios.
D: Lean Cuisine with tomato salad.
S: 1 scoop Chocolate Columbo fat free ice-cream.
Comments: Lazy day, didn't cook.
Exercise: 150 sit-ups *Great day!*

Monday

B: K-Time bar. *Need more food.*
S: Mandarin.
L: Big salad with tuna and 1/2 avocado, apple.
S: Box of sultanas and pineapple, yoghurt.
D: Steak with 2 oven-baked potatoes, heaps of steamed vegies.
S: 1 scoop Chocolate Columbo ice-cream.
Exercise: 150 sit-ups, 20 minutes on the treadmill.

Sum-up of the week

This person made great choices, had the right amount of treats and a manageable amount of alcohol. They need to work on taking the time to eat a proper breakfast though – cereal with yoghurt or a smoothie and cut down on the K-Time bars and biscuits – they should replace these things with fruit. Great healthy choice at fish markets. No surprises that this person lost two kilos in the first week. This is a brilliant food diary.

Across both of these diaries, each person needs to eat more fruit and more snacks. Remember, compare the food pyramid to your own daily intake and see where you need to eat more. For most women it is fruit, vegetables and dairy.

Most people have a big weight loss in the first week and then it settles down to about a kilo a week or less, depending on how focused you are and how much exercise you do. The rate at which you do it is totally up to you as long as you are happy with the progress you are making.

How much are you really eating?

One of the great things about the food diary is you can honestly see just how much you are eating. You may find that in between meals you're eating up to three or four snacks or that sometimes, for lunch, you may be eating two whole portion sizes. At night you might notice a constant pattern of comfort eating like the chocolate in Diary One. Once you discover how much you are eating you can really tackle your weight loss effectively.

Are you a grazer or a calorie thief? Grazing knowingly is one thing – whenever you get hungry, bored or emotional you shove something in your mouth. Some people graze all day, not because they are hungry but because that is what they have always done. Some people are like smokers and are addicted to doing something with their hands or used to putting something in their mouth all the time. If you are addicted to putting something in your mouth then grab chewing gum, sugar-free lollipops and sugar-free mints. I have become addicted to fruity lip-gloss. It feels like a treat, keeps me busy, smells nice and distracts me from wanting to eat when I am not really hungry. If you really must eat outside your snack time then have a piece of fruit. Also, try drinking water every time you feel like grazing. It can keep your hands busy and really curbs your hunger.

Calorie thieves dip into their kids' snacks or finish their sandwiches or eat what's left on their plate. Often, calorie thieves eat their extra food unconsciously. They also taste other people's food, test what they're cooking, and might find it hard to refuse food when it's offered to them. If you're a calorie thief, try to limit your eating to your meal/snack times. If you add up all the extras you eat you'll be shocked to see how much that adds up to during the week.

And don't forget that old classic: 'finishing your plate' syndrome. How many times did your mother tell you the starving kids in Africa story? If anything, that is reason enough not to overeat. You *don't* have to eat everything on your plate – learn to cook less or feed the scraps to the dog. There's always trouble if I leave leftovers uneaten or in my fridge, therefore I only ever cook enough for the meal; I don't plan for leftovers. If Kai and I are still hungry after dinner then we fill up on fruit afterwards.

Everything counts

Fifty excess calories every day may add up to a weight gain of 2 kg in a year. That's just three squares of chocolate a day. This means that with very little effort you can put on ten kilos in five years. That's how easily it happens. Just in case you don't see how much all those little things can negatively affect your weight loss I am going to spell it out for you:

- If you have three extra beers every night you can put on up to 20 kilos in one year.

- If you have one can of soft drink a day (on top of your calorie intake) you can put on 7 kilos in one year.
- If you have two chocolate biscuits every day (on top of your allowable fat intake) you can put on 4 kilos in one year.

None of it tastes so sweet, now, eh? *Everything* you do impacts on your life. Try to make the best choices that you can. Think of the outcome before you have a break-out. Knowing the consequences can help you stay focused. Just keep telling yourself: every little thing counts. Sure, every now and then it's good to treat yourself but not at every meal and not every day if you are trying to lose weight. Instead of treating yourself with food, make the choice to do some-thing nice for yourself like having a facial, a massage or having your nails done. For more ideas on how to nurture yourself, see Chapter 5 – Emotional Eating.

Water

I mentioned water earlier on but I need to tell you more. You need to start drinking water and lots of it. You need to drink at least a litre a day. Most people are dehydrated and don't even know it. Water is vital to our health and well-being. Without it our bodies struggle to function effectively. If you are hydrated properly your body will digest food more easily and will metabolise fat at a much higher rate. Water will help you lose weight.

You also need to start drinking water because once you start moving and exercising you are going to need even more to rehydrate yourself properly.

Drinking water has to become one of the habits you retain for the rest of your life. I found I never drank water, but now it's pretty much all I drink. At first it seems bland

and boring but eventually you will find it is the only thing that will fully quench your thirst. It does take time to get used to, but stick with it, as there are so many benefits.

- Water fills you up. If you have water before and after a meal, or in between meals, you are less likely to over-eat.
- You will fully absorb all the vitamins and minerals from food by being hydrated. The other plus is that as you are getting everything you need you are less likely to crave other foods.
- You metabolise fat (burn more calories) more effectively if you are not dehydrated.
- You may not be hungry, you may be dehydrated. If you are hungry outside a mealtime and have eaten your snacks, have two glasses of water and wait for your hunger to go away.
- As you get more active you need to drink more. You need to sweat to keep your body cool and if you are dehydrated before you start exercising you won't work as hard or burn as many calories. Drink before, during and after exercise.
- The more water you drink the less you will crave sugary substitutes.
- The more you drink the better your skin will look.
- The more you drink the better you will feel.
- By the time you are thirsty you are already dehydrated so it's important to keep topping up, all the time.

How to make water a habit
- Have a glass of water as soon as you wake up.
- Have a glass before you go to bed and have a bottle beside the bed.
- Before you reach for cordial or a coffee, have water instead.

- Use the water cooler at work or put a bottle of cool water in the fridge as cold drinks are sometimes more refreshing than at room temperature.
- Limit your caffeine and alcohol as they are diuretics and make you more dehydrated.
- When you do drink alcohol have water in between each alcoholic drink.
- Buy cartons of still spring water or get a water filter for home as the water tastes better and is easier to drink more of.
- Never run out. Always carry a bottle with you. That way you also eliminate having to make a choice.
- Have a drink of water with every meal. If you're still hungry, have another.
- Each time you open the fridge have a glass of water.
- Put an 'anchor' or notice in your kitchen reminding you to drink.
- Do it for long enough and it will become a habit.

Keep in mind that it takes twenty-one days to create a new habit and forty-five days to break an old one, so don't despair in your early days. The most important thing to focus on is what you are doing well and to simply keep going despite what you may or may not have achieved.

Snack effectively

Remember – snacking is not negotiable. You must do it at least twice if not three times a day. You *must* keep fuelling your body to encourage it to burn fat. You must snack with healthy food. Coffee, tea and hot chocolate do not count. You must eat food as well. If you don't eat enough snacks during the day then you will be starving at lunch or ravenous at dinnertime, make bad choices and probably eat too big a serve at the worst time of the day (particularly if it's dinner).

In order to snack well, don't run out of food at home. When you are hungry or starving you are less likely to be able to make a rational decision. You start craving comfort foods and nothing will stop you from having them. If you have to go out and buy something when you are hungry or starving, then chances are you are going to buy something very fatty and full of calories. I buy my fruit three times a week; and always before it runs out. I usually end up with a couple of brown bananas but I just throw them into breakfast smoothies or banana bread.

If you can learn to recognise this non-rational state of mind – craving – feed yourself immediately. Don't allow yourself to fantasise about what you could be eating. At lunch, if I am past my usual food time, I will stave off that out of control eating by having a yoghurt first, *then* make a decision about what or how much to eat. If I don't I will have two toasted sandwiches and while I'm waiting for them to cook, eat some lollies, not to mention what I might eat from the fridge when I'm looking in there for answers I'll never find.

With that in mind, *do not eat from the fridge or the packet.* Decide what you are going to eat, then go and get it. Presentation is everything. Take the right serving size, put it on a plate and sit down to eat it with a cup of tea or a glass of water. Your body is more likely to recognise that it's getting fed if you make a ritual of it. You also get the pleasure of focusing on your food. If you eat on the run you may eat more than you need.

Don't just have crackers, have crackers and tuna, or crackers and grapes. You don't have to go without to lose weight.

You just have to make better choices. Here are some healthy snack choices.

Rice crackers; Salada with Vegemite or light peanut butter; Rice Thins with sun dried tomato and tuna; boiled egg; celery and carrot with light dip; sultanas; fruit sticks; low fat muesli bars; crackers with dip; smoked salmon on pikelets with a dash of low fat cream cheese; Weight Watchers ice cream with fruit salad; Cadbury Diet chocolate mousse; dried fruit (apples, apricots, etc); Betty Crocker Low Fat Fudge Brownies; poached fruit; nuts – almonds, pistachios; fruit toast with low joule jam; skim milk smoothies; Vita Weets with tomato, lettuce, low fat cream cheese; Sun Rice Express Fat Free 3 Minute Noodles; protein bars; sushi; beef jerky; air popped popcorn; a cup of vegetable soup; low fat yoghurt; fruit salad; baked pretzels; crispbread with prawn and avocado; frozen mango; Special K bar; Space Food Sticks (only one at a time); Chuppa Chups (sugar free); canned peaches; jelly snakes; Arnotts Snack Right bars; K-Time Muffin Bars; Weight Watchers cookies; English muffin and low joule jam; slice of toast and small can baked beans; Freedom Foods Low Fat Corn Chips and salsa; Ski D'lite drinkable yoghurt; fruit, fruit, fruit, fruit or fruit.

Remember you should be having at least three pieces of fruit a day. And if you eat lollies you *must* have a piece of fruit or some yoghurt beforehand. Control those cravings by making sure you have filled up with something healthy as well.

Alcohol

And now for the bad news. Alcohol is an absolute killer for weight loss. It contains too many 'empty' calories that just don't get burned up. They add up, and you are more likely to eat more (and make bad choices) when you are drunk, and then everything falls apart when you are hung-over because you generally wind up having a fatty hangover breakfast. You have to keep drinking to a minimum. I go without during the week then have two to three glasses on the weekend. About once every two months I give myself permission to have a big night but usually wind up choosing to only have a few. The reality is if you really want to change your body for the better then alcohol really has to be significantly reduced. If that is a problem then you need to seek counselling (or go to Alcoholics Anonymous) because losing weight is hard enough (physically and emotionally) without being addicted to alcohol as well.

Shopping

Now you are armed with the knowledge of the kinds of foods you need to eat and how often you need to eat them, it's time to go shopping. Yes, I know that can be very scary. But don't panic. It's going to be OK. Just remember that low fat, low calorie food is the way to go. Check the nutrition panels in each product so you know what you are buying. Fresh fruit and veggies are fantastic, low fat dairy (milk, yoghurt, cheese) is great, wholemeal and high fibre foods are good for you, and lean cuts of meat will have you well on the way to your sexy new body.

Now, before you go out and get all this healthy food there are a few things you have to do:

1. *Eat. Do not shop when you are hungry.* I know you know it, but how often do you do it? You end up standing in the

confectionery section drooling over the Clinkers or pawing at the glass housing the cocktail franks. It's not a pretty sight.

2. Make a shopping list and stick to it.
3. Avoid the lolly aisle.
4. Go through confectionery-free checkouts.
5. Get someone else to shop for you or come with you.
6. Shop on the internet and avoid impulse purchases.
7. Don't stop at the bottle shop.
8. Don't go through the food hall first.
9. Don't stop at the ice cream shop on the way out.
10. Stay focused and remind yourself of your goals.

Summary

- Find out how much weight you need to lose
- Set a long-term goal for your weight-loss, then break it up into manageable chunks of time
- Buy a calorie counter, some low fat cookbooks, and use slimming magazines for extra inspiration
- Plan your meals a week ahead, and go shopping regularly
- Read the nutrition panels on packaged food to check fat units and calories
- Write your food diary – do it every day! And add up your fat and calorie intake
- Eat regularly: breakfast, snack, lunch, snack, dinner, snack
- Drink lots of water
- Cut back on alcohol
- Do your best and forgive yourself when you crumble.

Quick Quiz

1. At school:
   a) When it came to sport, you wore the mascot's suit and carried the water bottles on at half time.
   b) All the other kids called you Fatso so much that your teacher thought it was your surname.
   c) You represented the state in running, swimming, volleyball, basketball and hockey. You were also asked to do soccer, but you just couldn't fit it all in.

2. The last time you exercised:
   a) Olivia Newton John was asking you to get physical.
   b) Was while you were dreaming, and even that was fifteen years ago.
   c) Was an hour ago.

3. Sport:
   a) Is what you watch while eating fifteen pies and drinking a bucket of beer.
   b) Is wrestling your breasts into an 18 DD. It's like two sumos fighting their way inside a handkerchief.
   c) Is what you live and breathe for.

Mostly a: OK, so you got off to a bad start. It doesn't mean it has to stay that way for the rest of your life, though. And the mascot is an important part of the team's morale! I should know.

Mostly b: OK, no more watching sport, unless it's a replay of your team (yes, the team you *play* on) winning goals on the soccer field.

Mostly c: And you would be reading this book for what reason? Oh, your aunt's neighbour's second cousin is fat and you feel so sorry for her you thought you'd give this to her as a gift. Go away, please.

4

The Basics, Part Two

Shake your booty!

'I never ran a thousand miles. I could never have done that.
I ran one mile a thousand times.'
Stu Mittleman, World Record-holder
for ultra-distance marathon running

The reality is, if you don't start exercising you won't reach your weight loss goal – at least, not for a very, very long time. If you eat healthily but don't exercise you could expect to lose about 5 to 8 kilos in a year. However, if you exercise three to four times a week with the same healthy eating habits, you can lose up to 50 kilos in one year. That's the difference exercise makes – and it's a pretty big difference.

When I am in weight loss mode, in the course of a week I can play soccer twice, do one dance class, lift weights three times, swim once and run at least three times. I also go for 7 kilometre walks with my friends once or twice a week. I love doing most of it; sometimes the runs are hard and there are days when I don't want to do weights but I want a healthy body more, so I just do it. I know I will feel better and more energised afterwards. But the important thing is that most of the exercise I do is for fun, and is social. The soccer is more thrilling than anything I have ever done (see chapter 10 for details) – it's fun and leaves me with a great sense of self-esteem and achievement. I swim for relaxation while Kai has his swimming lessons, my walks are a great time for me to catch up with my friends, and I do my dance class for the sheer pleasure. When I dance I feel ten years younger and totally connected to my body; it reminds me of a time when I was carefree and my life held so much promise. I get in that dance room and am instantly transported. It pushes me both physically and mentally but when I leave I feel I am a whole foot taller. That feeling is priceless.

Running, though, is my real challenge. One day I want to run the entire City to Surf, from beginning to end – including Heartbreak Hill. It will be my coming of age, the time when I make a total transition from fat girl to fit chick. It is my Everest, really. These days I like to constantly push myself to do better. I don't always want to struggle through my runs, breathless and body tired, I want to do it with athletic ease. There is a great Nike slogan: 'If I can do this, I can do better' and it has become a mantra for me. I run every day but can only run 8 kilometres an hour; my current goal is 7 kilometres in 35 minutes. Each time I cut seconds off my time, and fall over at the end convinced I am dying of a heart attack, I remind myself that if I can do that, then I can do better. And one day I will cross that City to Surf finish line having run 14 kilometres in sixty minutes.

I do weight training to tone my body. Because I was obese, there was a lot of skin to lose, and I've still got the 'fadubadubas' (as Kath and Kim would call the floppy bits of your underarms). Kai often pats my underarms, assessing their development. 'Your fadubadubas are getting better, Mummy,' he says. That very honest feedback just fuels me to keep going. I love being muscly and strong but also want to have legs that are toned enough to carry off a mini skirt, one day. (But knowing my luck, by that time fashion will have swung back to pants!) The great thing about doing weights is that muscle burns fat by just being there in the body so if you've got good muscle tone, you're a natural fat burning machine.

If you are anything like I was (seriously obese) you should start off slowly with low impact exercise. Yes, I know you probably hate exercise. I hated exercise. Well . . . I *thought* I did. What I actually hated was being so fat that I couldn't exercise without severe discomfort, but I was so busy using Pluto Pups as a love substitute that I didn't know how good exercise would make me feel about myself – or the amazing things it would do to my body. Now, I live for going to the gym or playing a game of soccer. There is nothing more thrilling than chasing a girl half my age down the field, taking the ball off her, scoring a goal and winning the game for my team. OK, so that's mostly in my dreams but I *am* getting fitter, faster and better all the time, and I do score the odd goal. The endorphin rush I get from it is better than any drug I've tried.

Now, I'm not advocating that you throw yourself in the deep end and sign yourself up to everything and anything, with the plan to dominate the world championships in sprinting, marathon running and the 100 metres butterfly: the best advice I can give you is start slowly, try lots of different things until you find a few that you like, mix it up a bit so you don't get bored, and always push yourself a little bit harder each time you exercise. Before you know it, you will be fitter, happier – and losing weight.

The only way to burn fat from your body is to get your metabolism firing and to do this you have to eat regularly (which I've already covered in the last chapter) and move more, to get your heart pumping. You achieve this by doing what is called cardiovascular, or aerobic, exercise. Don't let the jargon intimidate you – it basically translates as getting your arse moving. If you increase your fitness, you increase the rate of calories your body burns. The more you move, the more you burn. It's so simple. Move more, lose more. If you keep saying that to yourself you will find it easier to do any kind of exercise. Another thing to keep in mind is the mantra 'bluff it till you become it' – if you just *do* it, eventually your body will demand it. You'll do it without even thinking.

When you start off you should do at least thirty minutes of aerobic exercise three times a week. As your fitness improves you should increase the time, amount and intensity of your workouts. I thoroughly recommend you join a gym as soon as you can. When you start, a gym instructor will show you the ropes and introduce you to low impact exercises, like walking on the treadmill, riding the cycle machines and doing light weights. Bit by bit work your way up to higher impact exercise by increasing the speed and time you exercise for (or heaviness of the weights). When you're ready, you can also have a crack at any of the exercise classes gyms offer – again, start slowly with lower impact classes like yoga or pilates, and work your way up to higher impact ones, like aerobics, Pump or Spinning.

If you are too embarrassed to join a gym at first there are lots of things you can do. Get yourself some low impact workout videos and do them every day, and walk, walk and walk until you are ready to take it up a notch. The key is to simply get started. There are things you can do without even leaving your home and things you can do without even getting off the couch. I started off with the simplest of exercises and slowly worked my way up. Now I run half marathons. Who would have thought? Definitely not me!

Here are a few things you can do to get started.

1. Bum squeeze
This can be done on the couch, in the shower, and at the check-out of the supermarket. Basically, what you do is imagine that

a twenty-cent piece has fallen in between your butt cheeks. Your job is to keep it from falling on the ground. Clench your bottom as hard as you can and keep squeezing for about twenty seconds. Let go, rest for ten seconds, and then do it all again. Do this exercise in sets of ten, and do as many as you can. I did them in front of the TV and now just do them whenever I am standing around waiting in a queue. It's great for the sexy, tight J.Lo bum you have always dreamed of having.

2. Tummy squeeze

This is great for achieving the flat tummy Brad Pitt is going to lick the whipped cream off. Sigh. Stand up straight and suck your tummy in as tightly as you can. Imagine Brad is walking by without Jennifer; try to impress him. Hold it in for twenty seconds. Relax for ten seconds and repeat as often as you can. Again, sets of ten are the best way to go. This exercise is like doing sit ups without the discomfort of having to get down on the floor (and if you've seen the mess in my house you'll know why I like these exercises).

3. Stair thingy

Find a step. If you don't have at least one at home then find a set of *Yellow Pages* and use those instead, or buy one of those kiddy steps. Stand in front of the step and step up and down ten times. Do three sets of ten, then rest for thirty seconds, and do it again. This is great for your bum and legs and should have you breathing hard. You can also give yourself the stair challenge. For one day a week do one set of ten on every flight of steps or stairs you walk up. Yes, people may stare at you but better that than the size of your bum, huh?

4. Sit-ups

Buy a fit ball and do sit-ups every day. If you do them in front of the TV those ads will benefit you more than they ever have before. If you don't have the room for a fit ball at home then do them on the floor, but get a yoga mat to make it a bit softer on your back. It's little things like this exercise that add up to make you make feel a whole lot better at the end of the day. Remember, every little thing counts!

5. Calf raises

You can do this exercise on your stairs or standing on some *Yellow Pages* while doing the washing up. Standing with feet slightly apart, lift yourself up onto the balls of your feet, hold for five seconds, then drop back down. You should feel a slight burning in your calf muscles; this will give you great definition in the legs.

When I started on my weight loss adventure I started with these basic exercises, then moved up to walking, then swimming and aquarobics. They were great to start with but ultimately I wasn't achieving the results I wanted. My heart rate needed to be at a level where my body would burn fat. Every bit of exercise you do is good for your overall health but some exercises are better for reducing your body fat. It wasn't until I started going to the gym and started jogging that the fat literally started melting from my body.

The best exercises you can do to burn fat are stair climbing, jogging, fast walking (otherwise known as power walking), aerobics, Spinning, boxing, rowing (in a gym at a fast speed and at high resistance), squash, soccer, Capoiera and dancing. If you're wondering what Capoeira is, it's similar to Latin dancing, but is mixed with martial arts, and all done to live drumming. It's *very* sexy and physically challenging.

The best exercises to tone and strengthen your body are pilates, Pump (weights), Body Balance, and yoga. Exercise that helps you maintain a healthy lifestyle but don't necessarily burn a great deal of fat are swimming, golf, friendly tennis, netball, aquarobics, slow walking, horse riding and casual cycling. Here's a breakdown, below, of some more calorie burners.

Light calorie burners	Moderate calorie burners	Heavy calorie burners
Casual walking	Brisk walking	Power walking
Casual cycling	Cycling up hills	Spinning
Gardening	Swimming	Heavy weights
Golf	Light weights	Judo/kickboxing/ karate
Tennis (social)	Squash	Football/soccer training
Housework	Football/soccer	
Yoga	Basketball	Stair climbing
Bowling	Volleyball	Cross-country skiing
Tai Chi	Skiing	
Aquarobics	Dancing	Aerobic dancing
Horseriding	Rock climbing	Advanced aquarobics
		Boxing
		Jogging/running

Note: The reason why there is a difference in the calorie-burning of a game of football/soccer and training is that during a game, activity is actually very stop-start. Training is constant activity, usually twice as long as a game, and generally involves high intensity fitness activity like sprinting.

For those who last exercised when leg warmers, sweat bands and Olivia Newton John were the height of fashion here is a quick guide to some popular exercise options you will find at gyms and fitness centres.

Aquarobics
Great if you are injured or need low impact exercise. If you are seriously obese, this is the start you need. It is gentle on

the body and if you do an advanced class you can actually burn a reasonable amount of calories. It is a series of repetitive exercises done in shallow or deep water (in deep water you wear a flotation belt). When I did aquarobics my only problem was finding a swimsuit to fit me, but I eventually lost about 20 kilos doing it, as well as swimming. The other 25 kilos I lost through cardiovascular exercise.

Body Sculpt

No, this is not liposuction! This is a very similar version of Pump, which is lifting weights to music, targeting different parts of your body.

Boxing/Body Attack

This is also one of my favourites, particularly if I'm feeling angry. There is no better way of getting your aggression out, especially if you are suffering from PMT. What you do is strap on boxing gloves and hit a trainer, the air or a punching bag. It feels so good to get through it. It gets my heart rate pumping and I feel strong, gutsy and invincible. God forbid that someone attempts to mug me after one of these classes – they'll get an uppercut they'll never forget!

Pilates

This is quite a slow, controlled class and works on your core strength and stability using props like straps to tone and strengthen your body. People rave about it transforming their bodies. It is great if you want a low impact workout.

Pump

This is also one of my favourite classes. This class helps you burn calories and tone your body. You use weights on a bar and a bench and work to a series of music tracks that have you targeting various parts of your body through the repetition of lifting light to moderate to heavy weights (depending on how heavily you stack your bar). It took me a while to enjoy it but now I lift more weight than the men and often find them stacking their weights on after they see what I intend to lift. *You* choose what level you do and the results can be seen in a matter of weeks. The advantages of Pump are that you have a whole class of people going through the same pain as you, and you have till the end of the music to finish what you are doing. I love what this class does to my biceps, legs and bum.

Spinning

This is one hell of a workout. It's one of the few classes that has me sweating buckets (and I rarely ever sweat!). It's certainly not what I thought it would be: I imagined myself with multi-coloured ribbons and lots of twirling around to Abba songs. Not so. It is stationary cycling at various resistances and speeds. You can adjust the speed and resistance yourself (i.e. cheat), but are inclined to work harder because the teacher is pushing you, and the rest of the class will see if you are going at a snail's pace.

Yoga

This works on so many levels – physically, emotionally and spiritually. I especially love Bikram yoga (where you do it in a room heated to 40 degrees) but it is not for everyone. There are many different kinds of yoga, so shop around and see what suits you. You don't have to be flexible to start (as most people think), because you become more and more flexible every time you do it. This was the only exercise that helped me get over the back injury I sustained when doing the splits in a nightclub (and believe it or not I was sober at the time!). It is generally low impact and can help alleviate stress in your day-to-day life.

Yogalates
This takes the best of both yoga and pilates.

Get the right equipment

OK, now that you've got an idea about the kinds of exercise you can do to get your new life on track, you need to get the right equipment. I'm not talking about a Thigh Buster from Danoz Direct – the first thing you'll need to buy is a good pair of running or walking shoes. Spend the money – your feet will appreciate it. Break them in slowly by wearing them around the house, then whenever you go shopping, then test them out on short walks. As they loosen up they will feel more comfortable, and only then should you wear them for a full work-out, power-walk or run. Think about getting orthopaedic inserts as well. They can really help if you're quite heavy.

The other thing you'll need to get is at least one very good sports bra. Buy two if you can so you're not always digging around in the laundry basket and doing special emergency washes. The bra is essential: the last thing you need is your breasts hanging down around your kneecaps. Invest in the support – it'll make exercising so much easier and more comfortable.

Burn fat

The best way to burn fat effectively is to exercise within what is called your 'target heart rate'. As I said, walking at a slow pace is good for your day-to-day health and well-being but it won't really help you lose weight. But don't panic – you don't need to work out to the point where you can no longer breathe, either. You just have to get your heart beating to a point where it goes into fat burning mode, which isn't as hard as it sounds.

To burn fat you need to work out to 60–80 per cent of your maximum heart rate.

This is easy to work this out. It is 220 minus your age. For example, if you are 35 years old, do the simple sum of 220 – 35 = 185 bpm (beats per minute). 185 is the maximum rate at which your heart should beat. Next, work out what is 60–80 per cent of that, and that figure is how many beats per minute your heart should be doing when you're exercising to burn fat. E.g. 60 per cent = 111 bpm, 70 per cent = 130 bpm, 80 per cent = 148 bpm. Being 35, I usually aim for working out at roughly 140 beats per minute. This has me slightly out of breath, still able to talk (only just) and sweating like a trooper. It's equal to a very fast walk or a medium-paced jog.

How do you find out what your actual heart rate is? The easiest thing to do is buy a heart rate monitor. It is basically an elasticised plastic strap that wraps around your ribs with a monitor (usually a watch) that shows you the readings of how long and/or hard you are working out. Some have timers, alarms and can even remind you if you drop below your target heart rate. (Use it when you do the housework and you will be pleasantly surprised how many calories you can burn.)

If you can't afford a monitor you have to stop exercising to work your heart-rate out, which can alter the reading a little. Find your pulse (on your neck or wrist) for ten seconds, count the beats and multiply by six. For example, 24 beats over ten seconds, 24 × 6 = 144 beats. 144 beats per minute puts me, at thirty-five years of age, at my best heart

Find your target heart rate

Age	50%	60%	70%	80%	90%	Max hr
16	102	122	143	163	184	204
17	102	122	142	162	183	203
18	101	121	141	162	182	202
19	101	121	141	161	181	201
20	100	120	140	160	180	200
21	100	119	139	159	179	199
22	99	119	139	158	178	198
23	99	118	138	158	177	197
24	98	118	137	157	176	196
25	98	117	137	156	176	195
26	97	116	136	155	175	194
27	97	116	135	154	174	193
28	96	115	134	154	173	192
29	96	115	134	153	172	191
30	95	114	133	152	171	190
31	95	113	132	151	170	189
32	94	113	132	150	169	188
33	94	112	131	150	168	187
34	93	112	130	149	167	186
35	93	111	130	148	167	185
36	92	110	129	147	166	184
37	92	110	128	146	165	183
38	91	109	127	146	164	182
39	91	109	127	145	163	181
40	90	108	126	144	162	180
41	90	107	125	143	161	179
42	89	107	125	142	160	178
43	89	106	124	142	159	177
44	88	106	123	141	158	176
45	88	105	123	140	158	175
46	87	104	122	139	157	174
47	87	104	121	138	156	173
48	86	103	120	138	155	172
49	86	103	120	137	154	171
50	85	102	119	136	153	170
51	85	101	118	135	152	169

Age	50%	60%	70%	80%	90%	Max hr
52	84	101	118	134	151	168
53	84	100	117	134	150	167
54	83	100	116	133	149	166
55	83	99	116	132	149	165
56	82	98	115	131	148	164
57	82	98	114	130	147	163
58	81	97	113	130	146	162
59	81	97	113	129	145	161
60	80	96	112	128	144	160
61	80	95	111	127	143	159
62	79	95	111	126	142	158
63	79	94	110	126	141	157
64	78	94	109	125	140	156
65	78	93	109	124	140	155
66	77	92	108	123	139	154
67	77	92	107	122	138	153
68	76	91	106	122	137	152
69	76	91	106	121	136	151
70	75	90	105	120	135	150

rate for burning fat (80 per cent). Here's a quick reference chart which shows you your ideal target heart rate for burning fat. Keep in mind that the bigger you are, the harder it is to exercise, so start at 60 per cent of your maximum heart rate, and work your way up. The only problem with finding your heart rate manually is that it is not 100 per cent accurate and you have to stop your exercise to get a reading, which in turn means your heart rate drops down, and your momentum has been interrupted. I reckon it's best to save up your take-away food money and buy a monitor – make sure you get one that is waterproof and that has a reading that tells you how many calories you have burned. Some gyms have monitors you can borrow to use during your workout, too.

Excuses, excuses, excuses!

'But I'm too fat to go to a gym!' – I used to say that all the time. And I can't tell you how many times I've heard, 'I'll lose some weight first then get to a gym.' Another popular excuse is also 'There's only skinny women in the gym.' But this is simply just not true – have a look around when you do actually get there; it's just full of normal, average-sized people getting fit. The most common excuse I hear, though, is, 'I don't have the time or money'.

I'm sorry, but there is no excuse other than the fact that you are not ready to do what it takes to lose the weight. If you order one take-away meal a week then you can afford a gym or fitness centre membership. You don't have to join the most glamorous gym and a lot of them have off-peak memberships at highly reduced rates. Many pools and leagues clubs have gyms attached and often they are a cheap alternative. If money really *is* an issue then just walk or run. That costs nothing.

You can find excuses not to exercise without any trouble. I used to say 'I'm a single mum, I haven't got any money, I don't have anyone to look after Kai, I don't like exercise, I don't have enough time.' But ultimately, it was simply my commitment to getting fit that I was missing. In the end I found the support, found the money, found the time and started loving the exercise.

If you truly want it to happen and are ready to do it then you will find everything you need to make it happen.

For example, you can become a morning person to find the time. I did – and sure, having a young child who has always been an early riser does help! I get up and get on the treadmill while Kai watches the cartoons in the morning. It's great bonding time and he is always hassling me for his turn afterwards. It's amazing the kind of person you can become if you truly desire the change. Remember – if you bluff it, you'll eventually become it.

Not enough money?

- Walking and running don't cost a thing.
- Pack your kids in a stroller and take them for a walk with you. If they're too old for the stroller, walk them to school every day. They'll benefit from the exercise as well.
- Walk with friends. Motivate each other to honour your commitment and to work a little bit harder every day.
- Give up one take-away meal a week and put the money into an off-peak membership to a gym.
- Approach a gym and offer to work in their crèche or to clean for a couple of hours in return for a membership.
- Hire a personal trainer only once every two months and get them to give you a training program you can do on your own at home or in a park.
- Hire a personal trainer and train with a friend, splitting the fee (make sure it is OK with the trainer first).
- Join a group sport team like soccer or netball. Put $10 a week away to save up for your registration (which generally covers insurance and your uniform). Once that is paid everything else is free. You generally train twice a week and play once a week and don't have to pay a cent more. You'll also work harder because if you have a coach like mine you'll have them yelling at you to run faster and work harder!
- Turn the radio up and dance with your kids for twenty minutes every afternoon.
- Buy some workout videos and do one every day.
- Take your kids to the park and run around the perimeter for thirty minutes.

Not enough time?

- Get up earlier.
- Stay up later.

- Use your lunchtime to go for a walk or go to the gym.
- Hire a treadmill (most fold out), weights and workout videos. Squeeze in your sessions whenever you have twenty or thirty minutes to spare.
- Use the stairs at work instead of taking the lift.
- Exercise while you watch the TV.
- Do some exercise while your kids are doing their sport or lessons.

Not enough support?

- Join, or form, a babysitters club. That way you simply 'pay' in time.
- If you are single, hook up with other singles. Parents Without Partners (contact details are at the back of this book) is a great place to start. Someone else may be looking for someone to look after their child. I formed a great relationship with a single mum and now our boys are the very best of friends.
- Join a gym with a crèche.
- Do a team sport with women your age and with your interests. I changed soccer clubs to play on a team who were all mums. The kids hang out together with one of the dads as mediator.
- Swim while your child has their lesson.
- Walk while your child does their ballet or gym class.
- Find a teenager you trust and pay them $8 an hour, one night a week, so you can get to the gym. The good thing is that they usually have heaps of friends more than happy to work for cash.
- Ask your child's friends over to play and encourage their parents to return the offer.
- Get a skipping rope and do it in your backyard while your kids are playing or sleeping. (Yes, the neighbours will

think you're mad but better to be mad than overweight and hating your body.)

- When the kids are asleep, run up and down the footpath outside your house. Short sprints at full speed for thirty minutes will have your metabolism firing on all cylinders.
- Get a punching bag. It's a great way to work out your frustrations while losing your bum.

If you do twenty minutes twice a day you have done your workout. Morning is best as it sets your metabolism burning all day, but whenever you can is better than never.

Bluff it until you become it

No one ever really *wants* to exercise . . . or maybe I should rephrase that. *I* never actually wanted to exercise – this was because the earth shook and my heart raced any time I actually got my fat bum off the lounge, usually to get myself another beer or Dial-a-Pizza. I never imagined there would be a day when I would actually *enjoy* running around on a soccer field. Although I do get a real kick when those endorphins hit me now, there are still many days when the last place I want to be is at the gym, or making myself run at seven in the morning.

Some days I really have to convince myself to go. When I'm finished it's a different story because I feel like Xena the Warrior Princess, but until that time I am still, mentally, the 110 kilogram girl who would much rather watch a rerun of Oprah than get on the treadmill or take part in a class that seems too hard to do.

What always gets me there, though, is remembering the kind of body I want, and the ways of tricking myself into working harder/running faster, or just getting to the gym in the first place.

First of all I remind myself of what I want: a healthy body. If I start coming up with excuses like 'I'm too fat for the gym', I remind myself that the only way out is through. Then if I am still trying to get out of it I make fake deals with myself. For example, when I do a Pump class I tell myself I will just work through the first three music tracks and then I can go and have a spa. When I get through those I tell myself I'll do just one more track, then one more and then another, until those endorphins kick in and I not only finish with heavier weights than anyone else but I get on the treadmill and run for twenty minutes after the class. This is how I bluff it until I become it.

When I started running it was the most unpleasant experience of my entire life (and this is the same person who has fallen down twenty stairs and completely destroyed her leg in the process). My breasts gave me black eyes, my recently-healed broken leg swelled up like a watermelon, my heart felt like it was trying to fight its way out of my chest and donate itself to science (not that science would have it), and all I could think of was getting my stomach stapled so I wouldn't have to do any more.

What got me through it was doing it slowly. I gave myself small goals – things I could definitely achieve – and slowly my fitness and strength improved. Now I run every day, despite being told twice in my life I would never run again. Bah humbug! I can do it, so can you.

When you go for a walk, set yourself a half-way point, and extend it a little bit more every day. Don't think about the return because you have to get back no matter how far you go (but keep the cab fare in your pocket just in case you don't!). Don't think about the bigger picture; don't concentrate on how hard it will be. Trick yourself into starting. Tell yourself you are going for a walk, and then walk most of it and run the rest.

For example, walk for four minutes, then run for one; then walk for four minutes and run for two.

Continually adjust your times as your fitness increases. I would set visual goals for myself, like, 'I'll just run to that tree', then, when I got there (if I was still able to breathe) I would extend it to a signpost, or where the track turned a corner. When I got out of breath, I simply walked until the Grim Reaper left the path. Then I started again.

If you run out of breath, don't just give up and tell yourself it's enough for the day. Recover, get your breath back, then try to push yourself a little further. Walk, or run, until you can't do any more, then recover again and keep going until you have exercised for the time you said you would. Instead of focusing on walking or running for forty minutes, I concentrated on the time until half way. I would say to myself 'only twenty minutes till turnaround', then ten minutes, then six minutes.

Another way of taking your mind off the work is to break up your walk or run; zig zag through the streets so you are going up and down hills constantly. Run down hills, as gravity is doing all the work. Take a different route every time, ensuring it never gets boring. Get yourself a Walkman so you can listen to music – just a cheap cassette or disc player will do. Put on your favourite upbeat tunes and be inspired by the music. I find I run faster and for longer if I have something to listen to. It's another good 'trick' to keep me motivated.

Set your time and do whatever you can to stay out. When I swam laps or went for runs I would stay until the time was over. On the days I was really tired or sore, I would walk or swim gently until the time was over. It's important to listen to your body, but if you are just being lazy then at least honour the time you said you would do. Never break a deal with yourself, because the only person who misses out is *you*.

Make your exercise a habit that is done on certain days. For example, Wednesdays become your walk day; Thursdays your swimming day and Saturday mornings are your Pump class. Write it in your diary. If it becomes a habit it is easier to commit to. Remember, exercise has to be a priority.

When it comes to exercise, you also have to constantly challenge yourself. Your body gets used to the exercise you do and becomes less effective at burning fat. The exercise you do when you're 110 kilos won't be nearly as effective at burning fat when you're 75 kilos. Keep pushing yourself. Run faster, run for longer, walk up hills, then run up hills. I know it sounds impossible now but if you start off slowly, then do a little more each time, you will be amazed at how quickly your fitness improves and how easily the weight drops off.

When I'm at the gym, I see so many women doing the same thing every day, reading *Who Weekly* and pedalling as if they are on one of those little paddleboats on the lake on a lazy Sunday afternoon (not that there's anything wrong with trashy mags – every girl needs to know what Paris Hilton was wearing last week). But in order to burn fat, you need to be sweating and slightly out of breath. On any of the machines at the gym, don't sit at a comfortable level for forty minutes, do thirty minutes and use all the levels. Work hard until you need to recover. Set the machine to 'Fat Burner' and be amazed at the great workout you get. Your heart rate will work at a much higher level and you will burn more fat than sitting there reading about whether or not J.Lo is getting married again.

Another good tip is to have lazy day exercises. We're all human, after all! When I don't feel like exercising I either go for a swim or take Kai for a walk. The important thing, though, is not to expect to become a world-class athlete overnight. Start off slowly and build your way up to more intensive workouts. Set smaller, achievable goals that will give you the taste of satisfaction and success. Setting unachievable goals simply sets you up for failure.

But even more importantly, when you are about to crumble, ask yourself if that is what you really want. Remind yourself that you will feel better if you make the healthy choice, remind yourself of your weight loss goal, and forgive yourself if you have a melt down or simply need a day off. Just don't let too much time pass, though, because it is always harder to restart.

Try and do a little each day, then do a little bit more. Always push yourself and acknowledge where you have come from rather than worrying about where you want to be. If you focus on the little steps, every step you take is closer to the person you want to be.

Shake your booty

- Go for a walk at least three times a week
- Just get moving – the more you move, the more you lose
- Make exercise a priority. Organise your life around it
- Wear good shoes, and a good bra
- Go for a walk
- Do something you enjoy, and do something new. Do it often
- Start slowly, then work harder and longer, bit by bit
- Find your target heart rate. Work to it
- Go for a walk
- Work as hard as you can, then work a little bit harder
- Find a friend to exercise with, join a gym or a pool, buy an exercise video
- Bluff it until you become it
- Go for a walk. Again.

Quick Quiz

1. Pluto Pups:
   a) Are the perfect substitute for boyfriends.
   b) Are the only reason you get out of bed in the mornings.
   c) Are evil.

2. Chocolate:
   a) Is the first thing you turn to when feeling sad, happy, angry, ecstatic, joyous, edgy or stressed. Anyone got a Freddo Frog?
   b) Chocolate: good. Vegetables: bad.
   c) Is not really your thing. You prefer to nibble on fruit, nuts and celery.

3. Food is:
   a) The most important thing in your life.
   b) Better than sex.
   c) Fuel. Next question, please, I've got four aerobics classes to get to.

Mostly a: You may need a little electro-shock therapy, but after a bit of work on yourself you won't crave food every moment of every day.

Mostly b: Keep reading. Everything's going to be all right . . . OK, maybe not, but keep reading anyway.

Mostly c: What are you doing here? Don't you have a nightclub to go to? Don't forget your hanky top. And don't forget your dinner – oops! – I mean, bottle of water.

5

Emotional Eating

Where the hard work begins

'I need to get back on track!'

There is no right or wrong track. There is
only one track – it's called living.

Hard work pays off

Even though I lost 45 kilos, the hardest work I did was
with my shrink Dr Nutcase. No amount of dieting had ever
taught me to eat and live healthily. Diets simply restricted
and controlled my food for a period of time where, certainly,
I lost weight, but as soon as I stopped, the fat would come
crashing back on because I returned to my bad old ways of
doing things. The truth is that I had to completely relearn
the way to live my life: I had to look at food differently, I had
to learn to respect my body and I had to learn to love myself.
I had to figure out *why* I craved BBQ Meat Lover's pizzas
and Pluto Pups in abundance. I had to come to the understanding that getting to a size 12 would not make me happy.
Ironically, making myself happy was what got me to a
size 12.

We know what it takes to lose weight: eating healthy food
and exercising. But if it is that simple why does Australia
have one of the highest rates of obesity in the world? I get so

many emails from women who say their story is exactly the same as mine: they eat in order to hide in their fat, then eat because they hate themselves for being so fat. Other women have been abused and continue the cycle of abuse by killing themselves with food. (Don't kid yourself – obesity can kill you.) If this sounds like you, I really can't recommend enough that you get a shrink, counsellor, therapist or support group to work through the reasons why you may be treating yourself this way. The only way to stop doing this to yourself is to look at why you are doing it, then find techniques to help you overcome your need to make bad decisions, and then learn to make better choices.

Once again there is no magic pill or potion, and no special incantation that will make you magically crave lettuce (I wish), but if you simply persist and stick at it, you will make important life-long changes. I never thought that, one day, McDonald's would no longer be attractive to me. I still do crave hot chips occasionally but I have much more of a handle on that behaviour these days; those thoughts are no longer all-consuming. I am on the way to being normal and healthy. It might take me the rest of my life to have it completely sorted out but I am light years away from where I was three years ago when I was morbidly obese and hating myself. I have committed to living healthily for the rest of my life now, accepting the good times with the bad – and let's face it, there will always be bad times!

Again, it's important to take it slowly, pick yourself up, wipe the cake crumbs from your mouth and just *keep going*. Do the very best you can, but when you stumble, forgive yourself, learn from it and move forward.

Why am I 'hungry'?

If something horrible happens to me my first impulse is to console myself with food or alcohol, or sometimes both. When I'm feeling low, I have to constantly work at not giving in. We eat for many reasons, not all of them hunger. Certain foods make you happy. For example, chocolate is a classic. It replicates the chemicals released in your brain when we are in love.

I crave hot chips because it's one of my 'happy' foods. Of course, they don't really make me happy, and usually make me unhappier than I was before I was craving them. I have to work on reminding myself that those foods no longer make me happy. I crave my particular happy foods because I associate them with good times in my life: every Friday night Dad would come home with a big bag of fish and chips, Mum would keep it warm in the oven and the smell would waft through the house. I remember it as one of the few times we were together and happy as a family. When I am distressed and seeking something to make me feel better, hot chips are one of the things I immediately think of, and then crave.

As time goes by I am getting better at not sabotaging my good work and hurting my body by overeating these foods but I am no saint and there are still days when I do give in. My cave-ins are down to about once every three months now, instead of three or four times a day when I was really unhappy. But I understand, now, that it was an addiction entrenched by years of abuse, and it may take many more to get it completely out of my head.

When I am craving food, especially hot chips, it usually means I am feeling stressed or unhappy. First I remind myself how I will feel after eating the hot chips. If I am still craving, I say out loud: 'Stop, AJ. You don't eat that way any more.

You make healthy choices. You deserve a healthy body.' Next I eat something healthy and then have a look at what I call my nurture list, and do something nice for myself, like having a facial, a bath, or painting my nails; or have a look at my distraction list, which is full of ideas just to keep me busy. If I'm *still* craving, then I make a date to actually have the hot chips, like the next Sunday after soccer. Of course, by this time the craving has gone. Otherwise, at crumble point, I cook myself a healthy baked potato, or wedges or whatever is closest to the food I'm craving. However, if I do end up crumbling, I eat the food and then just get on with healthy eating. It's important to avoid the 'Oh well, I've failed, so I might as well eat anything and everything' syndrome.

Learn to recognise what's going on in your life emotionally, and do whatever you can to avoid having a break-out. Nutcase calls it 'recognise, challenge, distract'. Recognise the old behaviour, challenge it with a new positive thought process and distract yourself with a healthy food or activity.

Here is my cravings action list:

1. I try to work out why I am craving the food. Identifying my feelings helps me solve the problem. I am usually feeling unhappy, stressed, unloved, unsuccessful. I also may just be feeling bored.

2. I remind myself how I will feel if I eat the food, and tell myself that it doesn't make me happy any more.

3. I picture a stop sign and repeat my pledge: 'I deserve a healthy body . . .' (see page xiv). Sometimes I go so far as saying out loud 'No, AJ. Don't do it.' Sometimes I write down 'Hot chips versus sexy red dress in three months time. What do you want more?', then read it out loud.

4. I eat something healthy, then look at either my nurture list and do something nice for myself, or my distraction list and just keep myself busy.

Healthy happy food

If you know there are certain foods you crave when you're feeling needy, make sure you have a back-up plan. Have food in the cupboard or freezer that can healthily replicate the food you are craving, thus avoiding a total crash and burn.

Fish and chips: You can buy low fat fish fillets from the freezer section of the supermarket; and cook healthy low fat wedges in the oven, using the tiniest spray of cooking oil.

Chocolate: Have a protein bar, like a Protein Plus Chocolate Fudge Brownie, or a Nestle Diet chocolate mousse with half a punnet of strawberries. Heaven!

Chocolate cake: Look for Betty Crocker Low Fat Fudge Brownies at the supermarket, and low fat chocolate muffins.

Chocolate milkshake: Using skim milk, have a protein shake like Aussie Bodies Chocolate Protein Revival, or use Cottees Diet Chocolate sauce and whizz up a smoothie.

Pluto Pup: Yes, you can buy low fat hot dogs. You can find them in the fridge section of the supermarket.

Hamburger: Make a home-made veggie hamburger using a lentil patty, a bun without butter or margarine, and lots of salad; or use extra-lean beef mince and grill it, again using the bun and lots of salad.

Pizza: Make a home-made low fat seafood pizza (see page 305).

Sweets and lollies: Substitute with licorice or jelly snakes.

Make your own healthy happy food list. Think about the foods you use to comfort yourself, list them, and then figure out a healthy replacement. Put this list on the fridge so that as soon as you go into that craving state and start fantasising about buying and eating certain foods, you can look at the list and go into immediate crash and burn avoidance.

If you actively work on these issues, I promise you, there will come a time in your life where eating healthily and living healthily is not an issue. I did it. So can you!

5. I avoid going near the shop, which stops me making a rash decision.
6. If I am still craving, I make a date to have the food at a later time, by which time the craving has passed.
7. If I am still craving after all this, I make myself a healthy alternative.

Nurture List

Every girl needs a nurture list. Mine works in two ways: it encourages me to do something nice for myself when I'm feeling down, which is particularly good if you've had a history of abuse or self-abuse (or not – it's good to nurture yourself anyway), and also works like a reward system for my good choices, like not giving in to the craving. (There's more on rewards later in this chapter.) I have a list of lots of different things; some take very little time and effort to do, and others involve spending quite a bit of time on myself. What I decide to do depends on how big my craving is, and how bad I feel.

Put your list somewhere you can see it, so that when you are stressed out and can't think properly, you can automatically look at the list and do at least one of those things to make you feel better. There's no room for thinking rationally when you are in tears, breaking plates or about to stuff chocolate cake in your mouth, so prepare for the moment so the moment doesn't bring you down.

The things on your list can be as simple as patting the dog, giving yourself a pedicure or having a bath, to having a weekend away from the kids – whatever will make you happy (and make sure it's not food, or related to food. Having a trip around the Sara Lee cake factory is not what I mean!). They need to be things that will cheer you up.

Here's mine:		Here's yours:
1. Patting dogs in pet shops	1.	_____
2. Picking flowers	2.	_____
3. Having a bath	3.	_____
4. Getting a manicure	4.	_____
5. Having a massage	5.	_____
6. Going to the races	6.	_____
7. Having a girls night out	7.	_____
8. Having a foot spa	8.	_____
9. Going for a swim and spa	9.	_____
10. Reading a book	10.	_____

Write your list, and stick it somewhere you will see it – on your mirror, a kitchen cupboard, or fridge – anywhere you can refer to it easily. If your work environment is what regularly sends you marching towards the fund-raiser chocolate, have the list in your wallet or purse. *Don't* contemplate drowning your sorrows in chocolate or alcohol, and especially not chocolate alcohol or alcoholic chocolate – do something nice for yourself instead. Oops. Need to stop talking about alcohol and chocolate. Think I need to refer to my own list. Back soon.

Ah, feel much better now. I really love the whole bath experience: candle, incense, soft music and apple juice in the wine glass (haven't I told you about that one yet? It's an alcohol substitute – looks the same, almost tastes the same, and in the right environment, works the same!). My baths are an easy escape hatch and give me time out to think about what is going on in my head. They immediately re-inspire me to keep working towards my goal. The more you can do these kinds of things for yourself when you're feeling down and about to lunge for the biscuits, the more they will become your new habits for life, and will help to keep you fit, healthy and happy for the rest of your new life.

Distraction list

This list is a bit different to the nurture list. I use this if I'm craving food and I just need to be distracted away from it. It may or may not be an emotion-based craving; it can be for a variety of different reasons, like boredom, boredom, habit, boredom and boredom. Either way, between the nurture list and the distraction list you need to recognise the behaviour, challenge it with a new positive thought process and distract yourself with a healthy activity.

Here's my distraction list:

1. Read a book
2. Go for a walk
3. Stick photos in albums
4. Clean out a drawer
5. Go window shopping
6. Write a letter to a friend
7. Update Kai's baby book
8. Surf the net
9. Condition my hair
10. Ring an old friend
11. Write a poem
12. Do sit ups
13. Paint Kai's wardrobe
14. Practise my poetry
15. Have a bubble bath
16. Give myself a mud mask
17. Write a comedy skit
18. File and paint my nails
19. Get a massage
20. Write a story for Kai
21. Sort out paperwork

And here's yours:

1. _____
2. _____
3. _____
4. _____
5. _____
6. _____
7. _____
8. _____
9. _____
10. _____
11. _____
12. _____
13. _____
14. _____
15. _____
16. _____
17. _____
18. _____
19. _____
20. _____
21. _____

22. Write my new book	22. _____
23. Write a song	23. _____
24. Go to an art gallery	24. _____
25. Go for a swim	25. _____
26. Eat a piece of fruit	26. _____
27. Organise the CD rack	27. _____
28. Give myself a foot spa	28. _____
29. Paint	29. _____
30. Make lurve.	30. _____

The reality is that breaking out with bad food choices when you're feeling depressed, stressed or just bored does not make you happy and very often makes you feel much worse than you did before. I remember feeling so disgusted with who I was that I would eat more to comfort myself about that awful feeling of failure. But when I learned to identify the disgust in the first place and why I felt it, I was able to take steps to make myself feel better instead of obliterating myself with food. Then I felt strong and proud for having made the right choice. It's important to note, though, that I'm not saying 'never eat chocolate' and 'never have hot dogs, Pluto Pups and pizza' – what I am saying is that you have to control the *amount* if you want to lose weight, and get healthy and fit.

Remember, no-one's perfect. I didn't have the will power of Cathy Freeman; in fact, I don't actually believe in will power. There were plenty of times I ended up chowing down on a Pluto Pup and chips like a rabid hyena, but I was also able to use what Nutcase taught me and learned from every experience. Whenever it happened I made a commitment to do a little bit better next time.

It's funny, really, I made a deal with myself that I would

not fully give up eating Pluto Pups. I decided I was allowed to have one each year at The Sydney Royal Easter Show, which is where this other 'happy' food of mine took its hold over me. For my family going to the Show was always a big, happy day out – one of the rare occasions we weren't all fighting and were actually glad to be with each other. Of course, Pluto Pups featured as the holy grail of family togetherness. Last year Kai and I went to the Show, and I'd been excited about having my legal Pluto Pup experience . . . but when I took the first bite, I was repulsed. Then Kai tried it and summed up exactly what I was thinking. He declared loudly, 'Yuck, that's disgusting!' I couldn't believe I had eaten so many and actually enjoyed them, or that I had dreamed so longingly of them. I'm glad to say that I'm now cured of Pluto Pups.

Thankfully, time moves on and we do evolve. Just because you can't imagine yourself living a healthy life with ease doesn't mean it won't happen. If it can happen to me – queen of the fast food outlet – it can happen to anyone. Even the laziest girl in the world can control her demons. It just takes persistence and the desire to change.

Stay calm

I could never understand those girls who say 'I'm so stressed I can't eat'. When I'm stressed I generally always over-eat. If day-to-day stress affects your eating habits you can deal with it pretty easily, as opposed to more serious eating disorders that have been developed to bury your emotions or avoid dealing with some serious childhood trauma. Day-to-day stress can be controlled, so be proactive. Get massages, take relaxing baths, do meditation or stress-control courses, learn to manage your time better and don't force yourself into situations where you are at the whim of other people's stress – it does rub off!

You may find that eating regularly keeps you less stressed. I know I get really cranky when I haven't eaten at the right time; as soon as I eat I am much more able to cope with whatever needs to be done. It you stick to the breakfast-snack-lunch-snack-dinner-snack regime you shouldn't ever get too hungry; and if you do, you know that a meal is never too far away. If you know you have a lot to achieve in a limited time, *be prepared*. Pre-plan your meals so there's no room for crashing and burning, take food with you where ever you go (and don't forget the ever-present water bottle), and take at least five to ten minutes to eat, so that you feel as though you *have* eaten.

If you make a commitment to being calm it will most definitely aid your weight loss. And if you don't support and look after yourself, who will?

Keep busy

Of course, on the other hand, boredom is a killer for eating when you are not actually hungry. Waiting for the movie to start at the cinema, sitting in front of the telly, or, if you are like me, endless hours at the cricket (yawn), can all make you start fantasising about what you could be eating. Tricky, isn't it? Well, not really; again, it's just a matter of being prepared. If you find yourself standing in front of the cupboard or fridge for no good reason, have a look at your distraction list and pick something else to do. If you recognise that you're just bored, and not hungry, you'll be more likely to make a good decision and stave off a crash and burn.

If you're sitting somewhere for a long time, beat the

boredom eating by keeping your hands busy. When I'm watching the telly, I give myself a foot spa, paint my nails, or give myself a mini-facial. Sometimes I even do sit-ups, just to keep busy. Take up knitting (Russell Crowe does it, you know!), or crocheting, or do some good old fashioned mending. Instead of constantly snacking in front of the TV, you can also chew gum or go for those great no fat, low sugar lollipops.

Another trick is to only have healthy snacks on hand so if you do have something it's low fat and does you little harm. This is great for when you're waiting for the movie to start – take a bag of pre-prepared fruit with you (grapes and strawberries are good) and a small bag of low fat, baked pretzels. If you absolutely must have popcorn, visit the supermarket before you go and buy air-popped popcorn (like Mother Earth Sundried Tomato) and a diet soft-drink to take in with you. Again, if you absolutely need an ice-cream for the 'whole' experience, there are all kinds of low fat frozen yoghurts and ice-creams that can do the same job as a choc-top.

If all else fails and you do have a boredom break-out, only eat half. Throw away the rest, tell yourself that it's OK and then make really healthy choices for the next few meals. Whatever you do, don't give up on yourself – remember the three steps forward, one step back theory. If you stick at it, you will get there.

That time of the month

Keep an eye out for pre-menstrual eating. I know it's not strictly emotional eating but it's not the best time of the month, is it? If you are anything like me you know you will have terrible mood swings, really big girlie outbursts, followed by tears and a hell tantrum, as well as the usual facial breakout, major bloat, painful days and nights and a general feeling of yuckiness. Oh, the price we pay to be able to breed!

I always crave greasy food, sweets and chocolate, and lots of carbohydrates when I'm either pre-menstrual or having my period. I try to be prepared by keeping a diary and marking the week before my period with a big red 'P' so I know that I'll be entering the premenstrual danger zone at that time. Before I was keeping track like this I would crash and burn every month and it was only when my period arrived that I realised what was going on. *Der!* These days I know it's coming up and I shop for it. I buy Healthy Choice 98% fat free frozen chips (for my hot chip/carbohydrate fix), I buy protein bars and Nestle Diet chocky mousses for the comfort food, and red licorice and Chupa-Chups for the sweet fix.

I also don't weigh myself before, during or after my period because it only ever sets me up for disaster: I always weigh 3 kilos heavier during my period. I would often weigh in, get depressed and then have a breakout because I had 'put on' weight and was feeling hormonal. Now I stay focused on my exercise and eating and look forward to a positive weigh-in the next week when my period is well and truly over.

Around this time it's important to keep up your exercise because you are more likely to binge or have a break-out. I always find the high I get from exercising helps me keep my eating focused, and the endorphins do fantastic things for my self-esteem. If you get cramps or just don't feel well at this time of the month, it's good to listen to your body and take it easy, so go for more gentle exercise like swimming, walking or aquarobics.

Reward system

'Finish your vegetables and you can have an ice cream', 'Have the needle and we can get some jelly beans from the doctor' – sound familiar? Your parents probably created this reward system and you are probably continuing what you have learned as a way of life. You have trained yourself to get rid of 'pain' by eating certain foods. How many times have you broken up with a boy and headed straight for the chocolate aisle? As we know, chocolate simulates the same chemicals in the brain as when you fall in love, which explains why I have spent so much time linking my fantasies of Brad Pitt with Chokito Bars . . . although I'm sure they don't even come close to measuring up against him (and we don't see Jennifer's bum bulging from too much chocky, do we?). The problem is we become addicted to it. We end up reaching for the Fruit 'n' Nut every day, and sometimes more than once.

If you eat chocolate or lollies every day it has to stop. Save chocolate as a reward only. How do you do this? Create your own, brand new reward system. Once a week, and only if you've been good for that full week, allow yourself to have one food item that you really love and lust after (preferably after exercise). You can have a piece of chocolate cake, a battered sav, a burger from Hungry Jack's – whatever it is you really love. I repeat, though, you have to have been good all week – this is a *reward* for your good behaviour. Also, it doesn't mean that you can say a bucket of fried chicken from KFC is one food item – keep it in perspective! You can also plot out a reward system for all your weight loss goals – from the first kilo, all the way to the final one. Write it up like a contract, and put it in your diary or on your fridge.

What will happen is the more weight you lose, the less attractive those food rewards will be. You eventually work out that you don't want to undo all the hard work you have done and are less likely to want those kinds of foods. When you get to this point, start replacing food with other rewards, like a facial for 5 kilos lost, and a manicure for 7, a weekend away at 10 kilos and a new dress at 15. Don't forget that you can also reward for centimetres lost off your body, too. If you are doing weights, you might not lose kilos but you will change shape. Reward yourself often, while teaching yourself that food is fuel only.

Start with the Good Week Deal. Set guidelines for the week that you must fulfil before you get your reward. Doing it this way means that, rather than looking at your week retrospectively, you can set clear goals for the week ahead and work towards your reward – it's a great motivator! You can also set one month deals, two month deals – you name it; if it works, do it.

Here is one of my Good Week Deals:

- Eat three pieces of fruit every day
- Drink 8 glasses of water every day
- Only drink alcohol one night, and then only have three drinks at the most
- Do cardio at least four times
- Do one session of weights
- Have no Coke, cake or hot chips
- Eat out only once this week and don't order dessert
- Don't miss any meals
- Only have lollies twice
- Cook myself a healthy low fat dinner three times

Reward: Get my nails done or have a Mint Patty.

Now plot the rest of your weight loss goals and rewards. Fill the list in, on the next page:

First kilo: _____

3 kilos: _____

5 kilos: _____

8 kilos: _____

One month deal: _____

10 cms off my body: _____

10 kilos: _____

Two months in The Alfalfa Zone: _____

15 kilos: _____

30 cms off my body: _____

20 kilos: _____

(and so on.) _____

Remember, though, that the reward system is based on being honest with yourself – if you don't fulfil your deal with yourself, you can't take the reward. However, it's important to set goals that are realistic and achievable, so that you are actually in reach of your reward and feel motivated to get there.

The best thing about rewarding yourself is that instead of focusing on the kilos you need to shift, you are motivating yourself to eat well, treating your body with love and respect and nurturing yourself all at the same time.

Heal your life

I buried my sadness in my eating and continued to do so until I buried myself in the copious layers of fat that surrounded my body. Then I was so unhappy with how out of touch with my feelings I had become that I ate more and more and more until I was numb – except for the mind-boggling self-hatred that swirled around inside my head a hundred times a day. Of course, not everyone who is overweight has been abused, and lots of people can avoid blowouts by managing the day-to-day stress in their lives. However, I get so many emails from women who *have* been abused in one form or another. It ranges from physical abuse, sexual abuse and paedophilia, to sexual harassment, domestic violence and rape. Some have lost one or more of their parents, partners, children and loved ones. I don't know what the statistics are but I know there are a lot of people out there overeating, or eating rubbish, or starving themselves to avoid dealing with pain from the past and moving into the future without the extra emotional baggage.

If this is your story, keep in mind that when you're beginning to face your demons, the idea is to forgive yourself, but never forget how you got there. I have no degree in psychiatry or psychology, and I don't think I could have achieved what I have without my Dr Nutcase, but I learned that no matter what happened to me, actually facing the pain and understanding why I felt it is the key to living with what happened and not being controlled by it. I say 'living with' because there may be painful things that you will never forget (and you shouldn't), but at least you'll know what those things are and that they are not remedied by abusing yourself with food.

Nutcase asked me to list all the things that had happened to me. Doing that made me realise why I felt so damaged and burdened. Then we actively worked on putting those things into perspective. One at a time, we broke down each painful event in my life. In the same way I worked at losing that enormous amount of weight, my emotional bigger picture was too big to tackle all at once, and so we took it one step at a time and allowed for set backs. Sure it was slow, but I finally hacked a pathway through my pain, suffering and self-abuse. Of course, I still hurt sometimes, but I know now that abusing myself with food isn't the answer to making it go away: making myself feel good in other ways is.

Understanding and accepting that I was not to blame for the abuse I suffered helped me to be kinder to myself. The bottom line is that you can't change the past but you do have control over your future, starting *now*. So don't let the abuse continue: find a psychiatrist, a psychologist, a therapist, or a support group – someone or something that can help you make sense of what has happened to you. Yes, it will be painful but if you learn to love yourself you will emerge stronger than you have ever been.

Learning to nurture myself through bad times without turning to food seemed like the magic potion I had been looking for but it took constant self-surveillance and a dedication to getting well. Remember, quick fixes like diets, laxative pills and simply not eating might have you losing weight (and only temporarily) but they won't make you healthy or happy, and they won't heal the pain in your life.

Here are some exercises that may help you on your way. They certainly helped me!

Why am I fat?

Make a list of the things you think have contributed (and still do) to your weight gain or unhealthy eating habits (other than eating bulk amounts of crap food – we already know that!). For example, here's some of mine:

1. I was abused by a teacher when I was a schoolgirl.
2. I was raped when I was seventeen.
3. When I was skinny I hated being harassed by men.
4. I stressed out when my mother died.
5. I feel rejected by my family.

Now write yours:

1. _____
2. _____
3. _____
4. _____
5. _____
6. _____
7. _____
8. _____
9. _____
10. _____

Why is being fat 'good' for me?

Make a list of the reasons why you think your weight, size or eating habits 'help' you. For example, here's mine:

1. Over-eating and bingeing distracts me from thinking about the past.
2. Being overweight makes me unattractive to men, therefore I am safe.
3. Food is my only friend.
4. Being overweight and 'out of control' is a convenient way of justifying negative thoughts, like 'no one loves me'.

Here's room for yours:

1. _____
2. _____
3. _____
4. _____
5. _____
6. _____
7. _____
8. _____

9. _____
10. _____

Why is being fat bad for me?

It's good to remind yourself of the negative consequences of what being overweight or obese are. Be honest and make that list – go on, no-one's watching. For example:

1. I am always tired.
2. I never go out.
3. I hate myself.
4. I don't get perved on.
5. I am killing myself.
6. I can never get clothes to fit me properly.
7. I only half live my life.

And here's room for yours:

1. _____
2. _____
3. _____
4. _____
5. _____
6. _____
7. _____
8. _____
9. _____
10. _____

How will being healthy help me?

Finally, make a list of how and why losing weight and getting fit can help you. For example:

1. I will feel sexy and fantastic.
2. I will feel powerful, strong and capable.

3. I will be fit and active.
4. I will live longer and be able to do more things, especially with Kai.
5. I will love my body.
6. I will get lots of attention but I will pick and choose whomever I want.
7. I will be in control.

And here's yours:

1. _____
2. _____
3. _____
4. _____
5. _____
6. _____
7. _____
8. _____
9. _____
10. _____

If you work on these lists (and doing them may take some time), you will start to see why you may have stacked on weight. With the help of a professional, you can go about resolving all those issues which may well be holding you back from reaching your goal weight.

Every time you feel like comforting or abusing yourself with food, refer to these lists. Imagine yourself healthy. Put yourself in that body and think about how good you are going to feel. Ask yourself where you want to be in three months' time. More often than not you will choose the healthy body option. If you do crumble and choose the unhealthy option, forgive yourself, but don't forget – analyse how you feel, write it down and read over it the next time you feel like you're about to go down. Remembering how a bad binge makes you feel will help you understand that food doesn't fix all your problems or make you happy. Only you can do that, from the inside.

I always say to myself that if I have enough time to drive to the shop and buy bad food, I also have enough time to talk myself out of it!

Bingeing and self-sabotage

As you will have figured out by now, bingeing can be a result of a few things; one is that you are using food to cover up pain. For me, though, another reason for my bingeing was when I went into sabotage mode. It almost always happened just before I was in reach of another weight-loss goal (99 kilos, 89 kilos, 79 kilos, etc). When I looked at why I binged I discovered that I was actually terrified of being thin. I wanted it desperately but was too afraid to get there. I would sabotage my good work with a big binge.

Nutcase asked me why I thought being thin would fix everything in my life and why I was waiting to be thin to start living my life healthily and happily. She made me sit down and write a list of what being fat and thin meant to me.

Here is what I came up with; fill in the blank list with your own defintions.

Fat is	Thin is	Fat is	Thin is
Unsuccessful	Successful	_____	
Ugly	Beauty	_____	
Abnormal	Normal	_____	
Unlovable	Loved	_____	

Not popular	Popular	_____
Lonely	Fulfilled	_____
Out of control	In control	_____
Powerless	Powerful	_____
Being judged	Not being judged	_____

I also felt that if I got thin, men might start harassing me again, and that I wouldn't feel safe, and also that I wouldn't have any more excuses to eat badly, over-eat or binge. In terms of my list, I should clarify that 'fat' is not all those things: they are simply descriptions of how I saw myself. Being overweight was just my excuse. When I took responsibility for how I felt, I didn't 'need' to carry the excess weight any more.

The crucial moment came for me when I referred to my list of 'thin' attributes – I realised I wasn't ready to be that person, I was afraid of being that person and I didn't really believe I could be that person. In reality, though, being thin had nothing to do with the fear I felt, and I had to lose 40 kilos before I understood that. I had to actively work on becoming that person before my body followed suit. This is where my 'bluff it until you become it' mantra came in handy: instead of thinking that all those 'thin' attributes would just magically flow into me once I lost the weight, I worked on making myself become that 'thin' person with the knowledge that if I did it for long enough, the behaviour would stick and I would become it whether I lost the weight or not. In the end, your goal should be to become healthy rather than be a certain size.

I put myself back in control by creating a safety zone for myself. Back in the bad old days there were many, many nights of stuffing endless amounts of chocolate, pizza, ice cream and cheesecake down my throat, trying to convince myself that a relationship hadn't worked because of the other person, not me; or because I was unloved and un-lovable because I couldn't maintain a relationship. I used to think that if I could just lose X amount of kilos I would never have relationship problems ever again. What I discovered with Nutcase was that I habitually gravitated towards people who could easily repeat the patterns of abuse I have known all my life. Now, instead of using my fat to protect me, I imagine a moat around my body and have some hard and fast rules about how and when I let people in. I only lower the drawbridge after a long time of getting to know someone. This gives me the luxury of keeping people who are bad for me out of my life; in turn this reduces the need to comfort-eat through sadness and loneliness.

I had really simple ground rules for this, like not rushing into relationships, telling people when to back off if they were invading my emotional space, being clear about whether I was interested in doing something or not, and refusing to be railroaded into an activity that would sabotage my emotional life or my weight loss. This was particularly good when friends or family tried to sabotage my weight loss by giving me chocolate or alcohol for gifts, or by bringing junk food into my house. I had to tell my friends that even though I valued our relationship, it was actually in danger if they couldn't respect and support the enormous commitment I was making to getting healthy. Some of those friends came with me and adapted to my new needs, but I also made new friends along the way. It's interesting, but sometimes the only thing you have in common with certain people may be an eating disorder, or an uncanny ability to drink three dozen beers between you!

I also made sure I didn't hang around with other binge

eaters and drinkers. I know these things sound really basic but they did make me feel safe and in control; I no longer needed the fat to 'protect' me.

I worked on being powerful and successful by working on a career-plan that would work. I became debt-free, I had business cards made up, I approached people for work, and I got it.

I also worked on no longer being lonely. I have always eaten more when I am single, feeling alone or in a relationship that isn't working. Food has always been my 'other partner' and I still have to work against that habit of thinking. To fill my life, I joined a soccer team and made so many friends my life transformed. I went out in big groups of women, which also helped me feel safe (you can see that safety – or feeling the lack of it – is one of my personal monsters). I forced myself to go to parties and gave my number to the people I wanted to get to know. Despite still being fat (but less and less so as the months passed) I was able to create the life I wanted. Being fat had simply been the excuse I used, like 'I don't have any friends because I'm fat', 'I can't get a better job because I am fat', 'I can't go dancing because I'm fat'. It changed to: 'I'm interesting and have a lot of people in my life', 'I go to lots of parties', 'I'm a great disco dancer and I love having tragic dance-offs' – let's be honest now, no-one does the moonwalk like I do! And one of the pluses in becoming a dancing queen is that you can burn a lot of calories – I'm sure I lost 5 kilos just by going night-clubbing. And there's nothing like skinny girls in tank tops to keep you focused on good food and exercise.

I also worked on being accepted. I spent time with people who loved and accepted me as I am, and cut contact from those who couldn't accept me, who put me down and made me feel bad. Accepting yourself and loving yourself as you are is probably one of the biggest things you can do when you're sorting through your emotional life. Realising that you can only ever be yourself makes the pettiness and unaccepting attitudes of others seem cruel, narrow-minded, elitist and pathetic. Remember, there are always people who will come into your life. Not all of them will or should stay. I used to blame myself and think that I wasn't good enough for people to love me or be friends with me. Now I look for new ways to keep busy and build my self-esteem, and tell myself it's the other person's problem if they don't want to know me, or can't accept me as I am, warts and all.

I'll never forget being stood up by a guy who later lectured me that the girl he married would have to be really special. The last words I graced him with were, 'Just because you can't see the beauty in everyone doesn't mean they aren't special. They are just not the right person for you.' (I think there was also a 'F**k you' as well, but that bit isn't as important!) If you are single and lonely, the universe may well be keeping you free for the right person – 'the glass is half full' idea is a powerful and positive way to look at life. But always remember, you are never going to find out if you sit at home eating chocolate cheesecakes! It's important to get out there, make a difference and challenge your old perceptions of yourself.

Have a look at your 'Thin' list. If 'beautiful' is on it, make sure you regularly feel beautiful by getting your hair done; having a pedicure; and shave your legs more than once a year. I seriously stopped looking after myself when I was obese, I no longer made the effort. I thought, no one else cared, so why should I? But you do care, don't you? You wouldn't be reading this if you didn't.

If you have 'successful' on your list then go out and do what it takes to be that – do a course, start up a business, get a better job. Think and act like a successful person until you become a successful person.

If you have 'popular' on your list then go out and join a group sport, class, interest group, have a party, say yes to everything you are invited to. If you act like the person you want to be when you are thin, you will be that person sooner than you think (and probably well before you get to your goal weight!).

Absolutes

Picture this: you manage to eat well for a week or two but then have a couple of days that aren't that great. You immediately decide that you have failed and that you will never get it right, so you give up and go back to bingeing to cover up the feelings of sadness and disappointment at not achieving your goals. Absolutes, or all or nothing thinking, is the very reason so many people (including myself) fail and continue to fail to lose weight for most of their lives. Back in the bad old days I would either be dieting, or failing at dieting; starving or bingeing; completely off alcohol or dancing naked on table tops having drunk the bar dry.

Thinking in this way will always bring you unstuck. This is why I say a little bit of everything is OK; there should be no forbidden foods and no banned substances, because the longer you go without something the more you will crave it. Whenever you have a crash and burn, don't give up – just get back into your healthy eating and exercise plan as soon as you can possibly manage it.

Just because you eat a piece of cake doesn't mean you're going to undo all the good work you've done and regain all the weight you've lost. Make sure you have only one piece, then make as many healthy choices as you can and follow it up with some exercise. Remember, even if you are taking one step back, you're also taking three steps forward. You'll be in front in the end.

I remember having a breakdown in front of Nutcase: I was devastated that I couldn't stop thinking about food all day, every day. I felt as though it was wearing me down and that it was proof that I had failed. Nutcase explained it all to me like this: when we ride a bicycle, which is something we all do with relative ease, we don't get on and think, 'I am holding the handle bars, I am now using the pedals, I am balancing and watching where I am going'. We only do this when we are learning to ride, but once we've figured it out, we simply get on and go. We only stop to think about it if there is something wrong.

It's the same when it comes to food and making healthy choices. When you are learning to eat well, you have to constantly remind yourself to do it, and it's not always successful. But after lots of repetition, not only will you be making lots and lots of healthy choices, eventually you won't need to think about it at all. You will just be doing it. Whenever you feel as though you have failed you need to remind yourself that you are learning, and that it's OK to ride into a few potholes. You might veer off course a little and get a few scraped knees, but if you just keep going, remind yourself of your goals and your pledge to yourself, you will do it. I did.

Learn to love your body

If you are using food as a substitute for love, learn to love your body instead. I found that the bigger I got, the less I loved myself, and the less I looked after myself. But as I lost weight and stopped using food as a replacement for love, I actually started loving myself more and treating my body with respect.

I discovered that if I took care of my body on every level I made important, positive connections with myself. The act of loving myself also made me want to be as healthy as I could be – it's a not-so-vicious cycle. Throw your heart into being happy; start a love affair with yourself. Give yourself a manicure and pedicure, get your feet back into shape with foot cream and pumice stones, polish your nails and make them look good. Every time you look at them you'll feel good about yourself. Moisturise your body; smother it with mango body butter, get in touch with it again. Shave your legs more than you do now, and wear dresses that flatter your shape. Wear your favourite perfume. Rediscover your sexuality, plan nights of love-making with your partner or boyfriend and make them really special with candles and music. The better you feel about yourself the less likely you are of sabotaging all your good work. Feel good and live well.

Whenever I looked in the mirror, I would often spiral into thoughts of despair. Even after months of hard work and good results, I'd still get depressed that I was still fat. Then I would crumble and eat rubbishy food that sabotaged my weight loss efforts. *Then* I would start in with all or nothing thinking, convincing myself that I would always be fat . . . and so I would go around and around in my self-destructive world of hopelessness. When I fronted up to Nutcase about this, she simply said 'Don't look at yourself in the mirror.' And believe it or not it was that simple. I stopped scrutinising what I didn't like and simply focused on living as healthily as I could. Just by doing that one little thing I cut out two or three binges a month.

Also, I would often think of speeding my weight loss up by skipping meals, or wanting to take diet pills or laxatives. I would catch myself thinking those thoughts and then repeat what Nutcase taught me. I would say out loud, 'I don't do that kind of thing any more. I am healthy and do not need to harm myself in that way. I love and respect my body.' Remember, taking it slowly is the only way you're going to come through this, and you need to take the time to enjoy and love yourself in the process.

Commit yourself

No, I'm not talking about sending yourself to the nuthouse, although I am surprised I never actually ended up there. I'm sure I've been close. What I'm talking about is making the commitment to being healthy, losing weight and doing it for the rest of your life.

Every single girl in the world probably has about three different dress sizes in her wardrobe. Even in *Sex and the City* the girls talk about having their 'skinny' jeans. I have a pair of these I am currently working my arse off to fit into. Skinny jeans are a great thing to have because they help keep you focused on your weight loss goals.

But what about the fat clothes? Why keep them? I'll never forget the day I threw out my fat clothes with gay abandon. That was the moment I decided I would never, ever allow myself to get that big again. In fact, I just threw out my very last 'goddess' dress – I gave it to another goddess. It was the first dress I bought (as a reward) after losing 15 kilos.

Letting go of that last goddess dress means that I'm making the final commitment: never needing it again. But I went a step further. I also threw out all the clothes I bought along the way. I dropped eight dress sizes so there was a reasonable amount of space created in my wardrobe (I feel a shopping spree coming on).

Don't keep your fat clothes. Make that long-term life commitment to yourself. It might sound kooky, but if you chuck them out when they don't fit you any more, you're making a very powerful, symbolic gesture. Each time you drop a dress size get rid of the evidence. And if your current clothes feel a little bit tight, get to the gym one more day a week, or look at your food diary with a magnifying glass and refine what you are eating. Whatever you do, don't dig out those big, comfy fat clothes. Don't make it possible to go back there.

Give your fat clothes to Vinnies. It was the only place I ever shopped when I was my biggest – now they can have them back!

There's a lot to learn

Apart from the amazing physical and nutritional changes you are making in your life, there will be a lot of change in your emotional life as well. There will be a lot more going on in your head than what actually goes into your mouth. I know I did most of my work intellectually and emotionally, and the support I received from Nutcase helped me keep working towards my goal.

I remember one of my melt-downs with Crusher, crying down the phone and wailing that I felt like I was being controlled. Crusher got very serious and told me something I have never forgotten. She explained to me that **I am in control.** I am the one who chooses to eat well and look after myself; I am the one who chooses to eat food that is of no benefit to me, or to miss meals or not exercise. No matter what the consequences are, **I am the one who is in control**.

This really made me sit up and take notice. I stopped crying that instant and realised that no matter what happened to me, it was up to me and me alone. Only I could do it; no-one else could do it for me. That moment of accepting the responsibility was an early turning point for me. No matter what has happened to you in the past, you are the only person who can be responsible for treating yourself well in the future. No one else controls what happens to your emotional life and body, except you. Simple, isn't it? But so true.

There is a lot to learn, and you won't learn it all at once. You have to try and try again. You are changing what Nutcase called 'learned behaviour', which can be anything from eating rubbish, bingeing, skipping meals, taking laxatives or a bit of everything. It doesn't matter what it is; it is something you may have done for most of your adult life, if not most of your life in general. When you find yourself about to act out this harmful learned behaviour, you need to take a moment and recognise that that behaviour is not good, nor is it welcome in your life any more. Then you need to remind yourself of what you are trying to achieve – 'I don't do that any more. I deserve better.' Visualise your healthy body, your active life. Finally, distract yourself with something that will make you feel better about yourself. Recognise, challenge, distract.

Understand that it takes time to learn these new ways of living your life. You have the rest of your life to do it, and anything you do in a positive way will benefit your health.

Deal with your emotional life

- Make a list of your 'happy foods' – the foods you find comfort in – and get them out of your home/workplace
- Find healthy alternatives to those happy foods, and get them into your home/workplace
- Write a nurture list, and use it
- Write a distraction list, pin it somewhere you will see it, and use it
- Stay calm
- Keep busy
- Mark in your diary when you are premenstrual and menstrual
- Plan your treats. Work out exactly what you will and won't allow yourself to have. Stick to it
- Write a time-line for your weight loss and your rewards
- Reward yourself often (preferably with something other than food)
- Get help – professional or personal. Whatever will work for you
- Do your homework: 'Why am I fat?', 'How does being fat help me?'
- Learn to love yourself
- Don't give up on yourself. Ever!

Quick Quiz

1. What does 'diet' mean to you?
   a) Diet is 'die' with a 't'. Been there, done it all. None of them have worked.
   b) Rabbit food.
   c) Nothing. Diets don't work.

2. Losing weight:
   a) Is for successful people.
   b) Is impossible unless I have shakes, diet pills, replacement bars, stomach stapling and my mouth sewn shut.
   c) Is easy to do. Just exercise and eat well.

3. Low GI is:
   a) That action figure I bought my kid for Christmas.
   b) The guy I have been stalking down at the Navy base.
   c) A great choice of food to help with weight loss.

Mostly a: Yep, there's definitely room for improvement. Keep reading . . . Please!

Mostly b: You should have a degree in failed dieting. You've probably tried diets no-one else knows about. It's time to start eating and moving – only then will you lose that butt of yours.

Mostly c: So when is your diet book coming out, smarty pants? You could probably teach me a thing or two.

6

The Six-week Crash

(And why diets don't work)

> 'We learn wisdom from failure much more than from success;
> we often discover what will do by finding out what will not do; and
> probably he who never made a mistake never made a discovery.'
>
> Samuel Smiles

Get off the diet merry-go-round

At the six week mark into my 'diet' I remember crashing and
burning, bingeing on four slices of Meat Lover's pizza, three
deep fried devil wings with ranch sauce and garlic bread, and
finishing it off with a huge episode on the phone to Crusher.
I just didn't think I could do it any more; I was bored and
wanted to feel 'normal' (whatever that was), instead of counting calories and fat and watching how much water I drank, or
obsessing about how much exercise I had or had not done.
Well, OK, I did have a broken leg at the time and the only
exercise I could do was on the bed and in my wheelchair, so
I'm sure my frustration levels were relatively high. But the
truth is, my broken leg wouldn't have made a difference
anyway: I would have hit that six-week crash and burn
regardless of whatever was going on around me.

Coming in at a close second to my 'Oh my god, I'm obese'
epiphany, that six-week crash was another huge turning point
for me. It was the day I figured out that healthy eating was a life

choice; that I wasn't 'on a diet'. After speaking to Crusher (who quietly, scarily, informed me I had no way of walking the food off, and that I should try to not do it again) I realised that I could never, ever return to my old eating habits – not without making a conscious decision to give up on myself once and for all, anyway. I laugh at that moment now, realising it was the day I actually broke up with Pizza Hut (they kept the pizzas, I lost my thighs). Now, a few years down the track, I may have put on a few kilos here and there for various reasons (some the result of things beyond my control and some the result of some self-sabotage) but I *know* I will never be obese again. I know this because healthy eating has become a habit and junk food is now very rare and not very satisfying any more.

It *is* that simple: successful weight loss is all about learning new habits. But why did my big crash and burn happen at six weeks? Well, it takes twenty-one days to break a habit and forty-five days to make a new one, so while I may have broken my old eating habits (like consistently eating bad food and overeating), I was still in the process of accepting new ones in their place (like choosing healthy food, understanding portion sizes and comforting myself with something other than food). I was in a weird kind of habit-learning limbo, and my brain did some sabotage because it just wanted to go back to its bad old ways. The great thing about the crash and burn, though, is that even though you feel like crap about it, you can learn from it and fine-tune what you're doing so that the new habits well and truly stick around for the rest of your life.

I've noticed that, at around the six-week mark, almost everyone I consult with at my weight loss club has a huge binge, starts putting weight back on, or has a really big boozy night out on the town, complete with the pigging out at three in the morning on hot dogs and pies. One person (I won't go into details, obviously) drank twenty-three beers, ate two pizzas, vomited, then ordered two more pizzas and ate those as well. This person has gone on to lose 23 kilos to date and only has a few more to go to reach their goal. My point is that crashing and burning at around this time is *normal*, even though it doesn't feel like it; you're missing your favourite foods, you're bored, edgy, no longer using food as comfort, possibly may be depressed and could even be freaking out about just how long it is going to take to lose the weight. Here are some other very common scenarios:

The creep crash and burn: Each week, bit by bit, you start returning to your old habits, like eating more and more take-away, eating chocolate every second day, or drinking a few more glasses of wine at dinner. At around the six week mark you have two or three days, or even a whole week or two, of making really bad choices.

The reward crash and burn: You reach a mini goal (say of five kilos) and then 'reward' yourself by eating like you used to with a big binge.

The plateau crash and burn: Everything has been going well, and you've been losing weight, but then it stops and it won't budge. You're angry, you think 'bugger it, it's not working', and throw in the towel with a 'fuck you' ('fuck who'?) binge.

The cold turkey crash and burn: You've been losing weight with a vengeance (and it's working), but it's boot camp. You haven't been treating yourself to nice things you can actually afford to eat, nor rewarding yourself, and you may also be missing meals, trying to speed your weight loss up. Bingo! You're bored (and hungry), and crash and burn.

And let's not forget the **I'm not good enough crash and burn:** Deep down inside you are either terrified of reaching your goal or don't actually believe that it's possible (in my case it was both). The only way through this is by constantly reminding yourself that you do want to get healthy, and to get some help (counselling).

With all of these scenarios (and there are as many as there are people trying to lose weight) the one common theme is not accepting that healthy eating habits are forever. While you can still treat yourself (and you must, if you are going to lose weight successfully and keep it off), eating 'normally' or eating like you used to is only ever going to take you back to your old weight and maybe even bigger than before. You have to be strong. If you have been overweight or obese you will *never* be able to eat whatever you want, whenever you want it – unless of course it's healthy, but even then you have to limit how much you put in your mouth. You need to take control.

Crashing and burning is like breaking up with your boyfriend and bumping into them a month later – before you know it, they're dribbling on your pillow and leaving their undies on your bedroom floor again. For some reason you have completely forgotten what a total bastard they were when they slept with the office redhead . . . and all her friends. So, why do we go back when we were so miserable? Because we are stupid? Well, no; it's because that behaviour is what we know and have become used to. It feels safe, even though it's not.

Forgive but don't forget

As I mentioned in the last chapter about emotional eating, the key is to learn from your crashes and burns. Remember how you feel after the event then remind yourself of that horrible, sickening feeling of failure just before you do it next time. Take some time out before you do anything, try and identify the real problem and remind yourself that that food won't make you happy (and that it may even make you feel worse). Return to your nurture or distraction lists. Remember: recognise, challenge, distract. Chances are you will choose not to binge or you will at least reduce the size of it. If it turns out that your binge is less than it would have been in the bad old days, then you are making progress. When I crumbled at that six-week mark Crusher actually made me realise I had come a long way from the binges of yesteryear: I had only eaten four slices of the pizza (as opposed to most of it) and I wasn't going to eat the leftovers for breakfast. Recognise the improvements you have made in your life rather than beating yourself up for 'failing'.

Also, remember what Nutcase called 'absolutes', in my last chapter? Just because you fall off the wagon doesn't mean it's all over, or that it's impossible. It's just life. It gets bumpy sometimes. You need to remind yourself that the sooner you get started on your recovery the sooner it will all be behind you.

A food conscience

Believe it or not, simply recognising that you are crashing and burning demonstrates that you have made progress. You have developed a food conscience. When you are constantly eating rubbish you numb yourself to what is going on around you and what is going in you; you just don't care at all. The thing is, though, you have already made a decision that eating badly is no longer what you want to do in the long term, and from that point onwards you suddenly understand the consequences of your actions and are taking responsibility for making choices, whatever they are – good or bad. So when you deliberately choose to eat something that is either full of fat, or two or three times the size you should be eating, of course you will feel guilt and remorse because you know this food is keeping you somewhere you don't want to be. But you are also very much aware of what you are doing. You're not on autopilot any more; and you're certainly not in Kansas any more, Toto. You have a food conscience. This is where your new life really begins. You are probably about to break up with junk forever, or at least only invite it round when it's right for you. Hallelujah!

Make the best choices, not just better ones

At this crucial stage of your new, admittedly bumpy, healthier life (and remember, it's better to have a bumpy beginning than a lumpy behind!), start thinking of your willpower as a defiant teenager, determined to do things their own way. You have to discipline it. *You* are the boss, *you* are in control, and *you* are the one who says it can't stay out past midnight. If you can survive the six week crash and burn (and any others that come knocking at your door) the next few weeks will be formative in creating new habits that will stay with you for the rest of your life. But you do have to start getting tougher on yourself. You've been making better choices all round, and you've been losing weight, but now you're going to have to start making the *best* choices in order to keep that weight loss going and get the results you want.

Before you move on to the next chapter on fine-tuning, I

want to remind you, again, that there are no quick fixes to losing weight. At around this time it'll be tempting to 'help' yourself along a bit. You may have lost a bit of weight already and your clothes are a bit loose. You hit the six-week freak out, think it's not working and start listening to the little devil telling you that if you go on a diet or use some quirky quick fix, and lose some weight fast, you'll eat healthily forever after that and won't have to go with this long, slow business. Well, this is rubbish. If this happens to you, you need to be prepared and understand what diets and quick fixes really do to you. Then you can get on with the serious business of fine-tuning and making the best choices with your eating and exercise.

Low carb/high protein

This is hailed mostly as the Atkins Diet. At the moment it's fashionable to subscribe to either all or part of this theory. If you hear people saying 'I don't have any carbohydrates after three pm', 'I cut out my carbs and I lost so much weight' or 'Carbs are the enemy' chances are they're doing this diet.

This diet is high in protein and high in fat, and very low in carbohydrates. The theory is that carbohydrates, which, when they are digested, convert to simple sugars in the body, increase blood sugar levels and trigger the production of insulin, which can increase the amount of fat stored in the body. Thus, anything with carbohydrates in them, from flour and sugar, and bread and pasta, to fruit and most vegetables, are not allowed. What you can eat though, is lots of protein and lots of fat, and non-carbohydrate based vegetables (that is, salad veggies). You tend to lose lots of weight quite rapidly on this diet.

You can have bacon and eggs, omelettes, steak, chicken – any protein – and you can cook it in fat, pretty much eat as much of it as you like, and you can have a bit of salad. Let's be honest, though, how long can you eat this kind of food for without getting bored? (Also, let's be *really* honest: the only thing that makes fat interesting is the carbohydrate attached to it.) Think about it: no bread, pasta, rice, fruit or substantial vegetables. Yes, the high fat foods do fill you up, but this diet is so limited that when you break out or give up altogether (and you will do either in all probability) your body goes back to the days of old and just stores everything as fat again. The failure rate on this diet must be sky high: you only need to eat carbohydrate and it's all over; you throw your body's finely-tuned new system into complete chaos. If you do start eating carbs again on top of the diet, you're actually eating a really unhealthy diet with the high protein and high fat . . . Bingo, you're back where you started again, and probably even fatter.

I'm sure pizza is like Vitamin C – without it you'll get scurvy and die (and seriously, you do actually need fruit like oranges to prevent scurvy). You also need lots of fibre to help with digestion, keep you regular, help with controlling cholesterol levels and prevent colon cancer, so leaving them out is not recommended, no matter how much weight you lose. And I reckon any diet that's high in fat isn't rational in the long term. I have heard this diet referred to as the 'halitosis and constipation' diet; in fact, one of the women's mags reckons that, after doing the diet to lose weight for *Cat Woman*, Halle Berry allegedly said she should have been called 'gas woman'.

What's the point in doing a diet like this if the weight comes rushing back on the minute you return to the foods you love? What's the point of being thin if you can't enjoy a bloody good bowl of pasta? Puhleeze! You just can't live like this for the rest of your life, and why would you want to?

Lose weight slowly and permanently and enjoy the odd hamburger, bowl of pasta and seafood pizza.

Prohibition doesn't work. If you really love something there is no point going without because you just set yourself up for failure. I love my carbohydrates, and couldn't live without them; in fact, I lost 45 kilos and still ate carbohydrates. I do watch my portion sizes, though, and I stick to the right amount of serves per day. The only time I eat more protein than normal is if I've done weights but otherwise, the key to my successful weight loss has been to keep food types variable and interesting enough to prevent boredom and keep me healthy, and to control my intake. Everything is OK and nothing is banned, as long as it stays within the general boundaries of my daily calorie and fat intakes.

The Zone
Again, like the low carb/high protein approach, this diet is all about regulating the body's insulin production, which in turn regulates the amount of fat that gets laid down in your body. This requires cooking regular meals, eating every four hours whether you are hungry or not, and is based on every meal having 40 per cent protein, 30 per cent carbohydrate and 30 per cent fat. All meals *must* contain low fat protein, carbohydrates, and monounsaturated fats like olive oil, and 75 per cent of each meal's carbohydrate must come from fruit and veggies. Not only does my head hurt trying to work this out, I think I'll have to go back to school and take advanced maths just to do the food shopping. It does use low GI carbs (glycaemic index – more on this later), which are good, and eating whether you are hungry or not is great for boosting your metabolism and staving off grazing or binges, but having to apply the food ratio to every meal is difficult and tedious to implement in the long term, I reckon. I went

through two pocket calculators trying to work out what I could have for breakfast – and by the time I gave my order to the waiter it was lunch time and the menu had changed!

Anything that isn't as simple as 'Take the Pluto Pup out of your mouth' just doesn't work for me. If I have to work out anything more than basic calories and fat, I head straight back to the freezer section of the supermarket where I can find the triple-chocolate-this-will-solve-your-life ice cream. Again, I think this kind of diet is high in prohibition and low in choice, so breakouts due to boredom and lack of variety are pretty likely to dump you back in a seedy, dark alley of Binge Central.

Liver Cleansing Diet
First up, alcohol is out, or not recommended, which immediately rules this diet out of my life as a long term lifestyle choice. So are dairy foods and foods high in starch (refined carbohydrates), fat and sugar; and protein is also quite thin on the ground as well. There is a fairly rigid eight-week schedule of eating which is two weeks of high raw veggies/fruit and low animal protein intake; followed by four weeks of pretty much vegetarian eating; followed by two weeks of high raw veggies/fruit and low animal protein intake again.

The idea is to kickstart sluggish livers, which in turn kickstarts sluggish metabolisms and thus helps the body rid itself of unecessary weight or fat. The diet also recommends taking nutritional supplements for calcium and iron (because the diet is low in dairy and protein), daily raw juices, and also a liver cleansing 'tonic', but there is no evidence to suggest that it actually assists in weight loss. You do need to eat lots of fresh fruit and veggies, which we all need to do, but you need to eat them raw as often as you can; there are some good pointers in the way of getting more legumes, grains, seeds and nuts into your life; and yes, no doubt it is good for you to cut the alcohol down in your life, but you can do that yourself with a bit more latitude than with this diet.

As I've mentioned, it's low in protein and calcium, both of which are essential for us, particularly as women (gotta watch the osteoporosis), and especially if you are doing weights, because you need protein to help build and repair muscle. Why be a slave to a strict diet and food plan and still have to take supplements because it's low on those levels? Everyone I know who has done it did feel healthier and lost weight but everyone put it all back on afterwards because in reality you can only stick it out for a little while. Even if you do last the full eight weeks, sure, you can continue the diet if you have more weight to lose, but why would you want to and still have a life? If you are an emotional eater, have a busy social life, or just like to have a drink and a packet of pretzels, you will almost always confuse the finely-tuned mechanisms the diet has put in place, go back to your bad old habits out of sheer boredom or frustration and then put the weight back on. And I can't even think about life without alcohol – not without having a drink first, anyway. Somebody pass the champers, please.

The Eat Right for Your Type Diet

This theory reckons that each particular blood group should have its own personalised diet; that certain blood types see certain foods as 'good' or 'bad', friend or foe. For example, Blood Type Os eat mostly protein and fat because they are similar to hunters and gatherers of prehistoric times (sounds like a few of my exes!). Blood Type As are similar to early farming communities and should eat mostly grains and carbohydrates. As Blood Type B is a mix of O and A, these lucky buggers get a mix of those food groups, as do those with AB blood. And yes, my head is spinning trying to figure this out, too. The problem is that if you are a Blood Type A but all your favourite foods are designated Blood Type O food, you are going to go without and eventually crash and burn unless you have a total blood transplant.

My blood type is AA and is yet to be added to this diet, but I have done some research and sent a letter to the creator giving him an outline of what is needed. Blood Type AA requires a diet high in champagne and Tim Tams. It works really well because AAs are never sober enough to realise their arses are so big they boast their own postcode. Seriously, though, I found the book very confusing. Like I said, 'Pluto Pup in, Pluto Pup out' works best for me, and will probably work the best for you, too. Strict regimes are *not* sustainable life choices, and being told what you can and can't eat just puts the brakes on the extremely interesting life you lead. It's far better to look at why you are eating three BBQ chickens for breakfast rather than becoming a food nazi. You just become boring and restricted.

The Bolivian Army Diet

This is also known as The Russian Army Diet and The Grapefruit Diet. It uses the same principle as the All Apple Diet, All Chicken Diet, All Soup Diet, All Egg Diet and All Tim Tam Diet: if you eat just one food for a certain amount of time you will apparently turn off it and reduce your portions of it in the future. (However, the theory behind the All Egg Diet is that after five days you will no longer have a social life and will never eat out, nor be invited anywhere ever again, thus eliminating choice . . . in anything.)

Obviously, these diets are all unsustainable. You can't live like this – as soon as you go out to dinner you've fallen off the wagon, and don't get me started on the excruciating boredom factor. You can't just have too much of one thing, it's just wrong in every sense of the word . . . Well, too much sex might be OK . . . Or money and sex . . . And maybe champagne . . . And naked men lying on the end of your bed . . . Too much of that is OK . . . But too much of anything else is just not realistic.

Now, for all my ranting about how diets don't work, there are, however, two general approaches that are good to look at to supplement your own freestyling weight loss and exercise plan. These are the CSIRO diet, following, and the low/high glycaemic index (GI) (next page).

The CSIRO Diet

First up, let me tell you that this diet was developed by the CSIRO with funding from the meat and livestock industry. It's a shame the nation's veggie and fruit industries don't have the organisation or the money to fund this kind of research. The CSIRO diet is actually quite a good eating plan. It's called the Total Wellbeing Diet and, not surprisingly, it is high in protein, but low in fat. It has quite a range of meal options but I'm not a big meat eater, so I would find the high meat protein element of the diet a bit challenging. Find it online at www.csiro.au. But as I said above, use the information to help you on your own way; add their ideas to your own method of what works and what doesn't. Use it as a very basic guide, and use the recipes (there's lots of great recipes, especially the soups), but there is nothing in the CSIRO diet that you can't do yourself with more flexibility.

The problem about being told what to eat is that it

doesn't allow for the emotional aspects of eating and eating out, and the importance of exercise. If you continually binge on certain foods or turn to foods for comfort, no food plan is ever going to keep you on track; no food plan ever gives you the flexibility for a spontaneous and interesting social life, and no food plan recognises that exercise is one hell of a big part of losing weight. Nothing works as well as learning to make healthy choices, finding good food you like to eat and learning to love an exercise that works for you.

Low/high GI

Low/high GI is not a diet, it's a measurement system of foods containing carbohydrates. 'GI' means 'glycaemic index'; 'glycaemic' means sugar or glucose in the blood, and the 'index' is a list of foods that contain carbohydrates which are rated on a scale of 0–100 depending on their ability to raise blood sugar levels. Foods that are digested quickly and rapidly increase blood sugar levels have higher GI scores, and those that are digested more slowly and raise blood sugar levels at a gentler, more consistent pace have lower GI scores.

Low GI foods tend to be more filling and give you a stable source of energy for longer, whereas high GI foods give you a quick fix and a 'spike' of energy but then leave you hungry a short time after (this is also known as a 'sugar low'). Obviously, when it comes to weight loss (and a healthy life in general), choosing lower GI foods helps meals last longer and stave off the sugar lows that lead to snacking and breakouts. For example, choose an apple over jelly snakes, yoghurt (low fat of course) instead of a blueberry muffin, and denser sourdough and rye, or less refined grain bread instead of highly processed white bread. These low GI foods will give you enough energy to get through the day without having to eat more or keep snacking until your next meal.

The Glycaemic Index is why I have my 'lolly rule': if I want to have lollies as a snack, I have to have a piece of low GI fruit or some low fat yoghurt first. I generally consider the GI factor of food when making some decisions (but not all): at breakfast, which has to last me until my mid-morning snack, and then at snack times because it has to last me till either lunch or dinner, when I will be very hungry. For example, one low GI breakfast choice is muesli, fruit and low fat yoghurt instead of jam on white toast, and snack choices are yoghurt, protein bars or fruit smoothies over processed muesli bars, sweet muffins or biscuits. There's more on low GI choices in the fine-tuning part of this chapter.

Buy a GI guide and read it at your leisure; it's better to be informed and incorporate as many helpful aspects of healthy eating without becoming obsessive about one particular way of eating. The University of Sydney has an excellent website at www.glycemicindex.com where you can search for foods and their ratings on the GI scale. But don't rely solely on the GI ratings of food to make good choices.

Quick fixes that don't 'fix' anything

And don't forget that the huge range of weight loss quick fixes out there are no substitute for a permanent change in your eating and exercise habits.

Starving yourself: If you start skipping meals or starving yourself there is no doubt you will lose weight – but you have to ask yourself, at what cost? Your body needs food for fuel, growth and healing, particularly if you are exercising, as well as for general immunity. If you skip meals or just stop eating, your body will start eating away at muscle because that's the first thing it does when it needs fuel and it's not getting it from a food source. It eats protein – your own lean muscle. Then, when you resume eating, your body has not only slowed down its metabolism, but it will be storing fat like there is no tomorrow . . . or I should say, like there is no meal tomorrow. If you keep up a steady supply of fuel, your body knows it's OK to burn fat. If you decide to skip meals or just stop eating to get there more quickly you'll only undo all the hard work you have done so far.

Here's a common scenario. You have a total crash and burn over your birthday, and put on a kilo (which is something that most people do if they love their food and have a few too many nights out celebrating). You panic because you've undone your good work, and go on a crash diet to get back to where you were. You lose three kilos, crash and burn again, put on two kilos, then eat only carrots and celery for a week, start skipping meals, lose one kilo, then crash and burn again and put on two kilos. Not only have you put on one kilo over four weeks but when you check your body fat levels, it has increased by five per cent. Why? Because your body has eaten muscle when you were in starvation mode, increasing your percentage of body fat and also started storing the food you did feed it as fat, because it didn't know when it was going to get its next decent meal. Instead, if you'd exercised and eaten well you could have lost between 2 and 4 kilos as well as 2–3 per cent body fat.

You can't just stop giving your body fuel. Feed it the right amount at the right times and you will steadily lose weight and keep it off, but if you don't feed it enough (or too much) it stores food as fat and puts the brakes on your metabolism. If you don't eat, of course you will lose weight, but you'll also lose your health – you put pressure on your heart and get palpitations, your liver goes into distress and you grow facial hair (to keep you warm because your metabolism isn't getting enough fuel to do the job). You also get bad breath and pimples, you lack energy and have not much resistance to illness. It's extremely glamorous.

One last thing: there's a difference between skipping meals to speed up weight loss and anorexia (and I condone neither), but if you feel compelled not to eat for any reason for a period of time, you are likely to have an eating disorder and need to seek professional help.

Purging: Yes, well, purging (or vomiting up the meal you've just eaten) is just wrong, obviously. Apart from always looking for excuses to leave the table, it's just not a good look coming back with carrot in your hair. If you are purging regularly, you have an eating disorder (bulimia) and need to get help. Don't ever throw up after a meal unless you have food poisoning. If you're running to the bathroom after every meal or 'bad' food choice you are not helping yourself at all in the long term. Sure, you don't ingest any fat or calories, but you are shirking your personal responsibility in terms of what you decide to put in your mouth. Not only will you receive no nutrients from the food you've eaten, you also lose essential minerals and nutrients in the process of chucking up. You can also develop either a loose or resistant gag response (which is dangerous for your health on both counts because you need a reliable gag response to prevent yourself from choking, when you need it), and you can also damage your teeth from all the acidic bile that is washing over them every time you upchuck. Another extremely glamorous quick fix (not).

Medical diet products: At the moment there is a medical diet product that you can only get by prescription from your doctor, which stops your body from absorbing about 30 per cent of the fat you eat. It costs a lot of money for each month's prescription, and in my opinion the way it works is highly unpleasant. It basically prevents the absorption of fat in your diet, and this undigested fat will pass through you, giving you fatty, oily (and smelly), liquid poo. For example, should you actually eat a meal high in fat it can cause you to have severe diarrhoea, you can also 'leak' the oily discharge and you can also have increased flatulence and/or abdominal pain.

Isn't it better to eat healthy food with limited fat and still enjoy the odd fatty meal, rather than rely on the discomfort and embarrassment of what might happen if you lash out? I think you'd be better off dealing with why you want this product to do such unpleasant things to you when you can achieve what it does much more pleasantly by yourself.

Laxatives: Again, another highly glamorous quick fix. Yes, laxatives will move any food you have eaten through your system very rapidly, but they can also strip the body of essential minerals, can cause liver damage and can increase the risk of colon cancer. Running to the toilet because you overate or feel guilty about what you ate is no way to live your life. If you are doing this it's likely you have an eating disorder because you are abusing yourself. You need to seek professional help.

Diet shakes/meal replacements: Don't fool yourself: these products are not food. As soon as you stop taking them and start eating 'normally' (that is, back to your old habits), the weight will come back on and you will have wasted a lot of money just to be back where you started. Shakes and meal replacements don't teach you new habits for life, and they don't let you enjoy the ritual of sitting down and having a meal and treating yourself well like a normal, healthy person. I just can't see the point. The only time I would use a shake would be if I was going out for dinner and wanted to fill the hole of hunger that would normally have me ordering the twelve-course degustation menu.

Slimming teas: These can reduce your hunger but why bother? You need to be hungry so you know when to eat. That's what healthy people do. If you are in weight-loss mode and are hungry before it is time to eat, drink some water, chew some gum, have a lollipop or a cup of black or herbal tea instead. If you think your hunger is controlling you and it drives you to distraction, then once again you should ask yourself why. Have you eaten enough? Have you had your snack? You should be eating every three or so hours in order to keep hunger at bay and keep your metabolism firing, so you shouldn't be hungry at any other time except just before your meal or snack. If you have eaten what you are supposed to but are still driven by the compulsion to eat then you need to look at why you are like this. No amount of slimming tea will help you in the long term.

Hunger suppressants/pseudoephedrine pills: In my humble opinion, these are basically legal speed. You can get heart palpitations and you can suffer from insomnia. I tried these and I found myself grinding my teeth, talking at 2000 words per minute (as opposed to my usual 1000), and could not sleep. They do reduce your appetite and apparently speed up your metabolism but so does eating regularly, and exercise, which also increases your strength, your heart-health, your energy levels, your self-esteem and your life. These products don't teach you how to live healthily and can cause you damage in the long term. And what happens when you stop taking them? Your hunger returns, along with all your bad habits, and so does the weight. Particularly with psuedo-ephedrine pills, don't let anyone tell you they are good for you. If you overdose they can cause seizures, heart attack and stroke. If a doctor tries to give you some as a dietary aid then I would think about getting a new doctor. They are not a long term, life changing solution.

Stomach stapling and liposuction: Hmm, let me think . . . Physically invasive, expensive and life-threatening medical procedures versus taking control of your life and losing weight healthily, happily and permanently. I know what I choose. To be honest, if you don't fix what's going on in your head, no amount of quick fixes will help you change your life or the way you feel about yourself. And if you really do want to lose weight with a vacuum hose, get off your fat bum and do the housework – it can count as a pretty vigorous workout.

Losing weight: If you have some kind of dark secret, hidden pain or acknowledged abuse in your life and are desperate to lose weight because you think it'll fix everything, I would suggest that losing weight is not the quick fix you're after. I used to think that being thin would solve everything in my life. For every ten kilos I lost I felt sure I would then live happily ever after, but it wasn't until Nutcase reminded me that when I was 43 kilos (and anorexic) I had still not been happy with my body or my life. I know it's a hard ask but you have to be happy in your body, no matter what size it is. Yes, be happy with the changes you make but don't expect the happiness fairy to land the day you hit your 'goal' weight. To lay on the heavy, hippy juice: happiness comes from within and being fat is the greatest distraction or excuse on earth.

So burn the diet books, and put the diet shakes, speed pills and meal replacement bars in the bin and get back on that weight loss horsey by cooking yourself a nice healthy stir-fry and going for a walk. If you lose weight slowly and consistently, you can have some fun without starving yourself or going without, and it's permanent. Remember though; you do need to put some controls in place, and you do need to be making the best choices from now on, but if you can just stick at it, and fine-tune, baby, fine-tune, you'll do it.

Stick at it

- Survive the six-week crash and burn
- If you do crash and burn, just pick yourself up, exercise and eat as healthily as you can
- Whatever you do, don't diet
- Stick with the food diary – make sure you're not falling back into bad habits, or the ways of old
- Reward yourself often
- Keep exercising. It'll keep your eating more focused
- Remember: no one is perfect. Just do the best you can.

Quick Quiz

1. What does 'control' mean to you?
   a) It's not that I don't have it – it's just that my stomach chooses not to use it.
   b) Sorry, what was that? I was too busy eating three hamburgers, ten Tim Tams and a packet of jelly snakes to hear what you were saying.
   c) Or do you mean 'restraint', or 'discipline'? Be specific. In five words or less. Come on, I haven't got all day.

2. During the day you will graze:
   a) On all leftovers from today's breakfast, yesterday's lunchboxes, last week's take-away Thai, and the chocolate cake you're just making – before it makes it to the oven.
   b) Your knees on the floor when you slip on those pesky lost M&Ms from last night's binge.
   c) On coffee, water, fresh air and cigarettes, followed by a box of laxatives and some home-grown mung beans, all before your daily four-hour workout.

3. My boyfriend:
   a) Loves me the size I am, but perves on size 8 women while offering me another slice of pizza.
   b) Is always honest about my dieting efforts. When I ask 'Does my bum look big in this?' he answers, 'Yes, would you like fries with that?'
   c) Checks the bin for Cherry Ripe wrappers hourly because 'he loves me'.

Mostly a: Here's a handy tip: don't go anywhere near the QE2 – you might end up being mistaken for it!

Mostly b: Put the lollies down and come with me. Remember, it's never too late to change your life.

Mostly c: All right, I think it's time you left now. There's nothing here for you, because we want to have our cake and eat it, too. PS: get some therapy.

7

Fine-tuning

How to get real results

'A goal is nothing more than a dream with a deadline.'
Joe L. Griffith

Overall healthy eating has begun to be a habit, you're really enjoying the new food you're eating, and the exercise is giving you a new lease on life. You're losing weight consistently each week and you feel great. However, soon you'll need to start fine-tuning your methods in order to keep the weight loss going. No-one ever eats a *perfect* diet, though; even top-notch athletes have different modes of eating – when they're in training, and out. But as I said in the last chapter, you can't get away with making only better choices if you want to keep getting those great weight loss results: you need to start making as many 'best' healthy choices as possible. When I am in fat-burning mode I try to make 90–95 per cent of my choices the best and healthiest. When I have a crash I just pick myself up and continue on, making sure the breakout doesn't go beyond one meal.

When you start your weight-loss lollopolooza, you'll probably see the weight drop off consistently each week after making a few vital changes in your day-to-day life. Also, when you start it's good to go for the things that will ease you into your new life – like trying to eat something for brekkie, cutting back on everyday fatty foods, chocky and takeaway and eating more healthy stuff, and doing some exercise – as long as it gets you on the weight loss train. The hardest part is getting started. But as your body loses weight, it gets harder to maintain that same consistent weight loss because as you weight less and less, your body needs less and less energy (from food) to get itself around, and you also need to start introducing more variety in order not to get bored. You need to start focusing a bit more in order to keep it going.

In your day-to-day activities you should be aiming for about 90 per cent of the best, healthiest choices. Go for the extra 5 per cent, too, if you can, but remember that you need to go easy on yourself; you can work up to 95 per cent over time (remember I've been doing this for a while now!) – make a commitment every week to getting a little bit better in your choices. Have a look at the box opposite, and notice the changes in food choices between the 'better' choices and 'best' choices. Keep in mind that these 'best' healthy choices should be sustainable for the rest of your life (with only a little bit more leeway for when you hit your goal weight), so don't be too stringent on yourself.

Remember, losing weight is a simple equation: input versus output. A 70-kilogram woman between eighteen and thirty-five years of age will burn an average of 2000 calories per day without doing any exercise. If you are on an eating plan of 1500 calories then you automatically burn 500 calories before you have exercised. Add to the mix a twenty-minute run (200 calories) or a one-hour brisk walk (300 calories) then you have made significant headway towards making permanent, healthy changes to your body. However, if you consume 2500 calories (which isn't that hard to do), your body is left with an extra 500 calories that it will simply store as fat. If you repeat this every day you are well on your

Better food choices	Best or ideal food choices
Breakfast	**Breakfast**
Special K Bar	Cereal, low fat milk and fruit
Low fat fruit smoothie	Low fat fruit smoothie and toast
Fruit and toast, with scraping of margarine	Toast, no margarine, fruit and low fat yoghurt
Toast, scraping of margarine, low calorie jam	Toast, no margarine, baked beans
	Fruit salad, low fat yoghurt, muesli
	Porridge and fruit
Snacks	**Snacks**
Muesli bar	Fruit
Jelly snakes	Protein bar
Up 'n' Go drink	Low fat fruit smoothie
Low fat biscuits or crackers	Rice cake with tuna
	Low fat yoghurt
Lunch	**Lunch**
Low fat Cup-a-Soup	Freshly made low fat veggie soup
Lean Cuisine	Protein salads e.g. tuna, chicken
Salad and meat sandwich with scraping of margarine	Salad and meat sandwich with no margarine
Dinner	**Dinner**
Lean Cuisine and veggies	Grilled fish and steamed veggies
Tinned soup and toast	Small bowl of pasta with tomato-based sauce and salad
Chicken satay stick and stir-fried veggies	Grilled chicken and salad

way to the land of lumpy thighs, of which I was queen, and believe me it's no place to live. The cost of living is too pricey.

Breakfast

Let's start with brekkie. As I have said, brekkie is a *must do*. Remember that old saying 'breakfast like a king, lunch like a prince and eat dinner like a pauper'? It's pretty much the truth. You need to eat breakfast because you have a kingdom to run – don't do it on a half-empty stomach. I know you've been resisting it (and I know all the excuses), but if you want to lose weight successfully, you have to eat, it needs to be something that's healthy, and it has to be within half an hour of waking (and I don't mean eating after half an hour of getting out of bed because on some days that could mean you've wasted three hours of potential fat burning). Don't wait until you get to work to eat, it's simply too long since you had your last meal. Get your metabolism fired up and give your body some fuel to get where you are going. Research has consistently shown that people who eat breakfast lose more weight, and keep it off, than people who don't.

So many people struggle with breakfast. A lot of my weight loss club members just make do by eating low fat muesli bars, or by having coffee and a piece of fruit, but it's not enough. I know those things are quick to do but so is making porridge (you can microwave it in less than two minutes and eat it in three), pouring some good natural muesli into a bowl with some low fat milk, and poaching an egg in the microwave to have on toast. Time is not an excuse. It's just habit: you've never made breakfast a priority. But this really has to change – and you need to be making the best breakfast choice you can if you're going to keep losing weight and make it stay it off. Fine-tune – it'll make a huge difference. In a little while you'll be waking up ravenous and will never understand how you ever got away without it.

I love breakfast time now. Kai and I sit down and have great chats before he heads off to pre-school. It is my special time with him. We make plans for the week and talk about what he's doing at kindy that day. We have spelling and counting lessons, and he's also learning that breakfast is a good and fun time. It also helps him focus on his eating and ensures he eats more than he would if I was running around the house, leaving him at the table on his own. People, particularly children, have more energy, concentrate and learn more if we have had a good breakfast. Give yourself (and your family, if you have one) the best start possible.

Eat something that will get you through to your mid-morning snack. Some muesli bars may be low in fat, but they are generally high in sugar (and have a high GI rating) so all they'll do is give you a quick burst of energy and leave you hungry before your snack time. You just don't need the added pressure of having to ignore hunger.

You might also need variety so you don't get bored. I am a creature of habit and have my cereal, toast and yoghurt on weekdays and have more interesting breakfasts that take longer to prepare on the weekend, but that works for me. If you're getting bored with your morning food, recognise it and look at other brekkies you can have – do some research, be proactive. Go through your cookbooks, your slimming magazines, get online. Find brekkies that you like and are going to last the distance on the energy stakes and *eat* them. It's amazing how quickly you become used to doing something different. You just have to do it for a few weeks, then you'll find yourself making better choices without even thinking about it.

Better breakfast options

Instead of having coffee and fruit or a muesli bar for breakfast have one of these instead:

- Small bowl of high fibre cereal with skim milk and a piece of fruit. (You could also try a bit of apple juice on your cereal – yum! Don't knock it until you try it.)
- 2 crumpets with Vegemite (no margarine or butter) and a piece of fruit or some low fat yoghurt
- 2 slices of fruit toast, low fat yoghurt and a small glass of juice
- 4 low fat pancakes with banana and maple syrup
- Porridge with banana and honey, made with skim milk
- Poached egg (1) on toast and yoghurt or a piece of fruit
- Scrambled egg (1) on toast with a small glass of juice
- 2 pieces of toast with low fat ricotta, and an apple to go
- Low fat/lean/lite bacon and 1 poached or scrambled egg on toast
- 1 English muffin with low calorie jam and low fat yoghurt
- Fruit salad, natural muesli and low fat yoghurt
- 2 pieces of toast with Vegemite (no margarine or butter), low fat yoghurt and strawberries
- 1-egg omelette and a piece of toast with low fat yoghurt
- 1 English muffin with low fat bacon and a grilled tomato
- Low fat banana smoothie and a piece of toast with Vegemite
- ½ pink grapefruit, 1 boiled egg and a piece of toast
- 2 slices toasted sourdough with lite peanut butter and a small glass of juice
- Stewed fruit compote with yoghurt and a piece of toast
- Small can of baked beans on 1 piece of toast and an orange.

Have a look at the list, above, of better breakfast options. When you've got into the habit of eating breakfasts like these, make your own combinations up – just make sure you're getting enough healthy food by checking the recommended servings on page 51, and keep an eye on your portion sizes (see page 162). Good combinations that will last you till snack time are: carbohydrate, fruit and dairy, or carbohydrate, protein and fruit. Also, there are so many high fibre cereals on the market it's just a matter of trying them to find the one you like the most. If you don't like one, don't give up – just move on to the next brand until you find one you do like. Just keep an eye on the sugar content, particularly those with dried fruits and honey, and always get the lowest in fat.

Lunch

After a few months in The Alfalfa Zone, you'll get bored with your lite ham and salad sandwich if that's what you're eating every day, so think ahead and plan your lunches when you do the shopping. Don't play it by ear and leave yourself open to bad food choices – I'm tempted to reach for fast, comfort food when I'm rushed off my feet and feeling a bit exhausted with the rest of the day ahead. So *be prepared*. Make pasta for dinner the night before and reheat it at lunchtime. Wrap up a few slices of your low-fat homemade seafood pizza from last night's dinner and take it to work with you. Above all, though, make sure you keep your food interesting, have it ready to eat, and again, watch your portion sizes.

Also, make sure you eat enough to get you through the rest of the day, or at least until your afternoon snack. Good choices for this time of the day are low GI foods like pasta (with low fat sauces), or big salads with tuna or skin-free chicken, or protein and/or vegetable based soups, and some fruit and/or yoghurt. You could also try having a desktop smorgasbord of, for example, baked beans, English muffin, yoghurt and a piece of fruit; or corn thins, low fat cheese, salad veggies and fruit. If you're out and about, it gets a bit trickier with all the choice you have at food courts, cafes and restaurants, but my next chapter 'Taking it to the streets' deals with this. There are stacks and stacks of low fat options these days so eating out shouldn't be a drama.

Dinner (learn to cook)

As I've mentioned before, I was the queen of take-away before I started to lose weight, and this really does have to be one of the changes you make in your day-to-day life, too, if you want to lose weight and keep it off. This means learning to cook. I know, I can hear you screaming, but it *will* fine-tune your weight loss. For breakfast and lunch you can get away with as little cooking as necessary and still lose weight, but dinner is usually where a lot of people come unstuck. It's the end of the day, you're tired; and what's more, at the beginning of your weight loss adventure you were able to eat a few takeaways and still lose weight, so you think you can keep doing it. But that weight loss will slow down and eventually stop if you keep it up. Remember – if you've lost weight already, your body needs less energy to get itself around, so it's even more important to focus on just how many calories and how much fat you are putting into it. Pull the veggies and beef out of the fridge and put on a bit of rice or a few noodles for the same kind of stir-fry you'd get at the Chinese takeaway but with fewer calories and fewer grams of fat. It's a hell of a lot cheaper, too.

Make time to look at your low fat cookbooks (especially the Women's Weekly ones; they're great), plan your dinners for at least a few days ahead and shop for them so that making dinner is easy. Leave the cookbook open on the kitchen bench for when you get home so you can make dinner straight away. If you're more of an unstructured person and like to make it up as you go along, make sure you have a healthy pantry and fridge, with enough of the right food groups ever-present so that you can whip up something quickly and easily. You can buy pre-cut and frozen veggies, and pre-cut lean meat like beef, chicken, lamb and pork at the supermarket these days, so there are no excuses in terms of not having enough time. And there are just so many fantastic low fat cookbooks out there now that you can cook the most amazingly tasty food. Food isn't boring – diets are, so make the investment and have a library of great cookbooks you can turn to every time.

Also, you might have been eating a lot of those fabby pre-packaged calorie-controlled frozen meals and bulking them up with salad or steamed veggies, but how long can you eat these for without getting bored and taking out a personal loan to cover the costs? Start cooking, baby! And when you do, stick with lean meats, low GI carbohydrates, fresh fruit and veggies. (Always keep a few Lean Cuisines on hand, though, for when you're too tired to cook and tempted to call Pizza Hut! You deserve better!)

A word on veggies

I know I bang on a lot about vegetables being rabbit food, but that's my problem. I had to learn to accept vegetables into my life, one at a time. If you're going to sustain your weight loss and keep it off, you need to learn to love these guys, too. They're terrific – they have no fat, and very low calories, most are low GI, and they actually burn more

Here are the best veggies for eating with little to no guilt:

- Asparagus
- Beans
- Beetroot
- Bok choy
- Broccoli
- Brussels sprouts
- Cabbage
- Capsicum
- Carrot
- Cauliflower
- Celery
- Corn on the cob
- Cucumber
- Eggplant
- Leek
- Lettuce (any kind)
- Mushrooms
- Onion
- Parsnip
- Peas
- Pumpkin
- Snow peas
- Spinach
- Tomato
- Turnips
- Zucchini

calories when you're digesting them than they have themselves, so eat 'em as much as you can.

Don't get turned off higher GI veggies like potatoes, though, just because of their higher blood sugar rating. Eat them too (they've got a lot of nutrients, or love, to give), but just keep an eye on your intake and calorie count.

Low GI foods

If you are looking to get longer-lasting energy from the food you eat, and I really do recommend this in order to keep those cravings and breakouts at bay, look at a GI guide to help with decisions about what food to eat. The veggies listed above, apart from potato, are low GI, so they're great. In terms of fruit, apples, citrus and stone-fruit are low GI, but tropical fruit like pineapple and watermelon are high GI. Also, avoid more refined foods made with white flour and sugar, like white bread, brown bread and cakes (obviously). Stick to mixed-grain, or whole-grain breads, sourdoughs and heavy rye, and wholemeal flour and pastas (also, cooking pasta till it's just 'al dente', or still a little chewy, lowers its GI rating).

Avoid rice like jasmine and calrose, and choose basmati or brown rice instead. Most processed cereals are high GI, so go for ones with rolled oats like natural muesli, and other high fibre brands that take longer to digest. Canned beans are good low GI choices (including baked beans) so you can add four-bean mixes (and others like it) to soups, salads and pasta recipes. I think I've banged on about low fat yoghurt being your new best friend, but it's also low GI, which is a great help. If you're after a lower GI option to starchy potatoes, use sweet potatoes or baby potatoes as they're lower in GI. Also, protein-based foods are lower GI, so lean meat, fish and eggs will fill you up and make you last longer too.

But as I said before, you don't need to live your life by the GI rating of food. Breakfast and lunch are good times to apply the low GI rule because those foods will get you through the day and/or through to your snacks. For me, snack time is good for low GI foods because they get me through to my main meals, so work out what works best for you. Another thing to keep in mind is that if you eat one low GI food in a meal, it will lower the rest of the meal's GI rating overall, so don't get hung up on making *every* ingredient in a meal low GI. Also, be very aware that 'low GI' doesn't mean low fat, so don't just eat a product because it says it's 'low GI': a lot of fatty foods are actually low GI because they fill you up and it takes longer to move through your system. The main culprits are chocolate, ice cream, and spreads like Nutella. Another myth is that wholemeal bread is low GI – it's not; even though wholemeal bread uses the whole grain, it's been highly processed and gets digested faster.

Cooking tips

When you throw yourself in to cooking, there are a few things you can do to help reduce your fat intake:

- always choose lean, 'heart-smart' or ultra-trim meats, or trim any visible fat from all cuts of meat
- buy skinless chicken like breasts and chicken thigh fillets. Chicken skin is full of saturated fat. Don't trust yourself to cut it off; make your environment safe by choosing skin-free at the supermarket.
- Don't fry food – steam it, stir-fry it, microwave it, grill it or bake it in the oven
- Use non-stick pans to cut down your oil use
- When you do need to use oil, use an olive oil or canola cooking spray, and use it sparingly
- Cook food in liquids like low fat stock, juice or water instead of oil
- Don't keep oil in the house (I don't) – you'll only be tempted to use it.
- Use low fat natural yoghurt instead of sour cream or thickeners (you can also use mashed potato to thicken sauces).
- You can buy low fat condensed and coconut milk, too, so there really is no excuse
- Use low fat salsas, chutneys and pestos instead of creamy sauces
- Use fresh herbs and spices to make food tasty, instead of butter or oil
- When using pre-made sauces only use a small amount and bump up the volume with water or low fat stock.

Know your fats

Remember, fat is stored as fat, so it's really important to go slow on any fat, 'good' and 'bad', unless you still want thighs the size of Texas. The 'good' fats are *monounsaturated*, and found in plant sources like avocado, canola oil, olives and olive oil, peanut oil, and certain nuts like almonds, cashews, pecans and peanuts; and *polyunsaturated*, found in cotton-seed oil, safflower oil, soybean oil, sunflower oil, certain nuts and seeds like walnuts, pumpkin and sunflower seeds, and omega-3 fatty acids found in some fish like sardines, salmon and tuna. These guys are good because they can improve your blood cholesterol levels.

'OK, great,' you're saying, 'I can eat some nuts and avocado, and cook with olive oil.' Yes, you can, but you should limit these fats to as absolute a minimum as you can – even though they're 'good' fats, they're still fat, and your body will still treat it the same way and slap it straight onto your fadubadubas if you eat too much of it. For example, a large avocado is 320 calories and 32 grams of fat. Nuts contain minerals, vitamins,

Don't go nuts

- 25 almonds (30 g) is 170 calories and 15 grams of fat (a quarter of your maximum daily intake).
- 12 cashews are 180 calories and 14 grams of fat
- 7 macadamia nuts are 200 calories and 21 grams of fat
- 15 walnuts are 185 calories and 16 grams of fat
- 30 roasted peanuts are 1990 calories and 16 grams of fat (yes, that's right, 1990 calories!).

protein, fibre and antioxidants but they still have to be kept to a minimum because of their fat content. I probably only have them two times a week at the most.

The really bad guys, though, are *saturated* and *trans* fats. If you keep eating these in any regular kind of way you certainly won't lose weight. Not only do these fellas decide to sit around your body like couch potatoes, both these fats bump up your 'bad' blood cholesterol levels; the trans fats in particular can do quite a lot of damage by bumping up your 'good' *and* 'bad' cholesterol levels. You can find saturated fats in food like full cream milk, butter, cheese, ice-cream, fatty red meat, chocolate, coconuts, palm oil and chicken skin. Trans fats are everywhere but manufacturers don't have to itemise them on nutrition panels so watch out for anything that has 'hydrogenated' in it, like 'hydrogenated vegetable oil'. A lot of packaged and processed food (particularly snack food and margarines), and fast food (like hot chips or fries) contain or are cooked in trans fats.

Know your marketing

- 'Fat free' food has less than 0.15% per 100 g
- 'Low fat' food has 3% fat (or less) per 100 g, and 1.5% fat (or less) in a liquid
- '98% fat free' food can only have 2% (or less) fat per 100 g
- '97% fat free' food can only have 3% (or less) fat per 100 g
- 'Reduced fat' food contains 25% less fat than the regular product, which doesn't necessarily mean it's low in fat, especially if the regular product is 98% lard.
- Any food with 7–15% fat per 100 g is a moderately fatty food, and anything with above 15% fat per 100 g is a high fat food. Avoid these ones.

Don't get too caught up in all this, though; the general rule of thumb should be to eat the good fats, the monounsaturated and polyunsaturated ones, like avocado, nuts and olive oil *sparingly* and try to avoid the saturated and trans fats as much as you possibly can. With this in mind, you can cook with olive oil cooking spray, use a canola or olive oil based spread for your toast and sandwiches (if you really need it), choose lean and low fat or 'heart smart' meat, particularly beef and chicken (always choose skin-free chicken) and low fat or reduced fat milk, cheese, yoghurt and ice cream.

Watch the sodium

Sodium is found in salt and too much of it can make you retain fluid, which is no good on the scales. It's generally good to cut it right down as part of a healthy diet anyway because it can put pressure on your kidneys and contribute to high blood pressure. Cut it out as much as possible or use lite salt instead. Always choose 'reduced salt' or 'no added salt' options when you're food shopping. Also, drink lots of

---

See ya, salt

- Choose reduced salt varieties of packaged food, like baked beans, tomato paste, bread, breakfast cereals
- Don't automatically salt your food, taste it first. Use herbs, lemon juice or the tiniest spray of olive oil to flavour your food in just as interesting ways
- Avoid salt-laden processed foods like powdered instant soup, instant pasta with flavouring, and watch your soy sauce and tomato sauce for the salt content.

water. It helps flush the sodium from your system and reduce fluid retention.

Portion control

As you lose weight your weight loss may become a little stubborn, but it's generally nothing a little focused eating can't fix. Your portion sizes can creep up before you realise. Misjudging your portions is also no good for your body's understanding of 'fullness' – research has shown that if you eat over-large meals, your stomach capacity can increase too, which then increases the amount of food you need to eat before you feel full. So keep your portion sizes under control. Have a look back at the recommended serves of food on page 51 to make sure you're getting enough of the right kinds of food, and then fine-tune your portions by checking out the basics following.

Your dinner plate: Split your dinner plate into four quarters. One quarter should be protein, another quarter should be carbohydrate and the rest (one half of your plate) should be vegetables. Make sure you don't over-stack it and don't go back for seconds.

Crockery in general: Don't use those ridiculously sized restaurant style plates and bowls at home. If you reduce the size of your plate, the correctly portioned size of your meal will look bigger and more satisfying.

The palm index: This is an easy way of measuring whether you have the right portion of meat. Any red meat portion should be no bigger than the size of the palm of your hand; a chicken fillet or breast can extend to the first knuckle of your fingers; and fish can be the size of your hand (all the way to the tips of your fingers). A huge rump steak or T-bone the size of an A4 page is definitely a no-no. In any case, you should be aiming for around 100–120 grams of lean beef or lamb; about 140 grams of lean chicken or pork; about 200 grams of lean white fish (less for the oilier fish like salmon and tuna); and about 100 grams of tofu.

Other recommendations: For breakfast cereals, think 'small bowl'. This works out to be about 45 grams of high fibre cereal, 30 grams of raw porridge oats, or about 50 grams of natural muesli. 'One serve' of bread is generally two slices of more processed bread or a whole English muffin, but it depends on the kind of bread – if the bread is heavier, like sourdough, it has more calories, so you can treat one slice as one serve. In terms of pasta, a good serving size is, for example, 100 grams of dry spaghetti. The whole packet is generally 500 grams, so you just need to portion away one fifth of it. For spirals or elbow noodles, about a cup of cooked noodles is the right serving size. About ¾ of a cup of cooked rice is generally what you should be having at any given meal. Try not to have more than 30–40 grams of reduced fat cheese, and keep the low fat yoghurt portions to about 100 ml (which is half the regular-sized tub!) For fruit, in general choose fist sized apples, small bananas and medium sized oranges. The bigger the piece of fruit, the higher its calorie count.

Eating out: If eating lunch in a café take the top off your focaccia or bun and only eat half the bread they serve. If dining out, stick to one course, or just order an entrée sized meal, and have a piece of bread. There's more on this in the next chapter, 'Taking it to the Streets'.

Eating up: Don't fall into the trap of telling yourself 'Well, I've exercised, I can eat more'. Studies have shown that women who exercise have a higher chance of putting on weight than men who exercise. Sounds silly, doesn't it? But post-exercise I am ravenous and have to be very controlled about what I eat, otherwise I eat for three. Planning your meal before the exercise will help you through this. If you 'eat up' after exercise then you may not put on any weight at all but you won't lose any either: you'll probably just maintain the same weight. Stick to your correct portion sizes and eat a piece of fruit twenty minutes after your meal if you are still hungry.

Eat at your meal time

If you are nibbling or grazing when you're cooking, and eating your kids' leftovers, then you're sabotaging your weight loss. If this goes unchecked, over time your intake will creep up and at the end of each day you could be eating the equivalent of three or four snacks instead of two, or two dinners instead of one. This kind of grazing tends to happen in the late afternoon or early evening, so avoid these situations by having a double snack. Snack at around your normal afternoon snack time, then again just before you cook dinner, or cook your children's dinner. Make sure that this second snack is fruit only, though – no excuses!

If you are eating enough during the day, and sticking to the meal/snack/meal/snack/meal/snack way of doing things, you really shouldn't be getting hungry until about half an hour before your meal or snack time. If you do feel 'hungry', it's probably just a compulsion to eat. We all love food; and it's played a significant role in our lives (I would never have reached 110 kilos without it). This might never change, but now I'm aware of the difference between my genuine hunger and my desire to eat. Once I recognise this I go into damage control depending on the severity of the cravings.

If it is close to mealtime then simply distract yourself till then. Look at your distraction list and do something that saps your attention until the time passes: jump on the internet, read a book, fold some washing, go for a walk, or if you're at work do something that you've been putting off. At the very least stop everything and have a glass of water, or make yourself a cup of tea.

If you are still hungry after your meal, have another glass of water and wait. It takes about twenty minutes for your body to recognise that it's been fed and is not hungry any more, so just hold off. If you're still hungry after twenty minutes, have a piece of fruit and count it as your post-dinner snack.

Hidden calories

	Calories	Fat (g)
Leftover child's peanut butter sandwich	80	5
2 fish fingers	130	5
3 cocktail franks	180	15
1 piece of brie (30 g)	90	9
1 slice of BBQ Meat Lover's Pizza	225	12.5
30 g roasted peanuts	190	16
2 bites of hamburger	105	4
2 leftover chicken nuggets	100	6
2 bites of a chocolate bar	115	5
1 chocolate biscuit	100	5
2 bites of ice-cream cone	35	2
A few fries from your child's takeaway	60	3
A handful of chips	60	4
5 squares of chocolate	160	9

In the box on the previous page is a handy load of information about grazing on snacks and consuming hidden calories that'll probably make you cringe. If you eat all this over a week (and it's pretty easy to do if you're not focused) you could be consuming approximately 1663 calories and 104.5 grams of fat. That's roughly an extra one or two day's worth of food. Not so tasty now, eh?

Slow down

I love food, and I love the process of eating. No kidding! I have plenty of photographic evidence and the stretch marks to prove it. I will always love food and the rituals that surround it. Even though I don't depend on food to make me happy or to suppress my emotions any more I still recognise that I really enjoy the process of eating. If I quickly scoff my lunch down in less than two minutes while I am working on the computer or playing with Kai then I usually find I still crave food afterwards. I may not be hungry but I want to eat more.

If this happens I know that what I am missing is the ritual of eating. I usually make a point of making my meal, presenting it on a plate, sitting down at the table and eating it, slowly, so that I enjoy every bit of it. I also get a glass of water and turn some music on. I make sure I acknowledge the meal I am eating – that way I am less likely to crave more food afterwards.

It's important to notice the difference between still feeling 'hungry' and not having satisfied your needs. Take your time when you're eating so that you don't overeat, but more importantly, take the time to *enjoy* the meal. Take pleasure in it. This is why grazing from packets of food or straight from the fridge is not very satisfying. You are like a pig at a trough, hurriedly eating anything in front of you, rather than taking the time and effort to savour what you have chosen to eat.

Do the same thing with your snacks. Instead of eating your apple in ten seconds flat, cut it up and and arrange it on a plate, get yourself a glass of water and some ice to keep it nice and chilly, put your yoghurt in a bowl with some fresh strawberries. At dinner time, make it special by setting the table with the 'good' plates and cutlery, put soft lighting on, have some water in a wine glass (or apple juice, or a small amount of wine), and put some soft, groovy music on. Make eating an experience that satisfies all your other needs, as well as your hunger.

Plan to let loose

Now, as I'm sure you've worked out from this book so far, eating salads and drinking water is not living in my books. If it was I would never have been able to double for Roseanne Barr. But having said that, you do have to plan your time to let loose. I never continued diets because I always thought I was going to have to go without beer, wine and Pluto Pups forever. Then I learned that there is a time and place for everything and moderation is the key to a healthy lifestyle. Personally I'd rather be a size twelve and enjoy my wine than be a tee-totalling size ten. Remember, this is the lazy girl's guide!

If you're going to go out for a drink, plan for it: have 'lean' calorie and 'lean' fat days on the lead-up to that night and on the days following. Make sure you do some extra exercise as well. Alcohol is full of 'empty calories' because it has nothing going for it nutritionally, but just because you're going out one night doesn't mean you have to blow your weight loss; it's just a matter of thinking ahead. The trick is not to drink

Here are some tips for managing big nights

- Make sure you eat before you drink. When I broke my leg I was completely pissed because I had made the extremely wise (not!) decision to save calories by not eating. If you don't eat, you'll get pissed very quickly and we all know what happens then . . .
- Make every second drink a glass of water
- If you're drinking wine, have a spritzer (half wine, half soda water or mineral water)
- Try not to mix your drinks. It'll end in a disastrous hangover.
- Beer, wine and creamy cocktails are killers in terms of calories and fat, so go slow on them or try and avoid them
- Spirits, diluted with diet mixers, like vodka and soda, and gin and soda, are probably the best choices in terms of keeping the calories to a minimum. I recommend Archer's Spri
- When you get home, drink lots of water, and make sure you've got water on your bedside table
- Don't have anything in your pantry or fridge that will tempt you to have the midnight munchies
- Plan your post-drink brekkie beforehand and make sure you've got all the ingredients you need at home so you don't rush out to the shops and get distracted by the hot chip shop
- Good low-fat post-drink brekkies can be a poached egg on toast with low fat bacon and some grilled tomato and mushrooms, or baked beans on toast and low fat bacon with the tomato and mushrooms, or just a low fat bacon toasted sarnie with tomato and mushies on the side. Not that I'd know, of course!

so much that you lose control and eat everything in sight, or that you drink so much you have the most heinous hangover the next morning (and/or break your leg falling down the stairs) and *then* eat everything in sight.

If you're a chocoholic, again, plan for your indulgences.

Don't cut it out; you'll only binge on it because you're not allowed to have it. Work chocolate into your reward system for kilos lost, or your good week deals, or keep a mental list of the low fat chocolate you can afford to eat: like Betty Crocker Low Fat Fudge Brownies, low fat hot chocolate drinks like Cadbury's and Jarrah, low fat chocolate ice-cream, Nestle Diet Chocolate Mousse Desserts (and there are stacks of other low fat chocolate products out there) or simply go for very high cocoa solids chocolate, which is just so rich you can only have a little bit. One person I know actually builds chocolate into her weekly food diary (indulging once a week on a certain amount), and has to tick it off at the end of the week.

Sports waters, cordials, drinks, juice

Beware! All of these things can skyrocket your calorie intake for the day. Make sure you read the nutrition information before consuming more than you should. Don't overdose on them, particularly juices. There's been an enormous proliferation of juice bars recently, and the bad news is that juice is really high in fructose, or the sugar found in fruit, so keep an eye on your calorie intake. Here are some interesting figures for you to look at:

- Gatorade is 110 calories per bottle
- Aquaveta is only 70 calories per bottle but if you have three a day you are drinking extra calories you have to burn off
- Ribena is 125 calories per cup
- Regular Coke is 105 calories per cup
- Regular Fanta is 135 calories per cup
- Hot chocolate from a café is 160 calories per cup
- A lot of the sparkling mineral waters with 'juice' are all around the 100 calorie mark per cup (150 calories per can).

The lesson here is to beware of those hidden extra calories. I only ever have sports drinks after soccer and I generally try to stick to drinking a small glass of juice in the morning and water throughout the day. If you must have cordial or soft drink make sure it is 'diet', otherwise train yourself to drink water.

Sugar and honey

Like alcohol, sugar and honey are empty calories which do very little for you and add up faster than you can imagine. If you have two teaspoons of sugar in your coffee or tea you are adding 40 calories to your tally; and two teaspoons of honey is 35 calories. If you are having five cups of tea or coffee a day you are going to have to work off an extra 200 calories for sugar, or 165 for honey, otherwise it'll get stored as fat.

There are plenty of sugar substitutes at the supermarket. When cooking things like cakes and slices, use Splenda powder as it measures cup for cup.

Be aware that there is also a high level of sugar in jams, sauces, flavoured milk, canned fruit in syrup, lollies, biscuits, jelly, ice cream and some breakfast cereals. By all means have honey on your toast (with no margarine or butter, of course) but don't add it, or sugar, to tea, coffee, hot chocolate, cereal or porridge. At least, not five times a day anyway.

Treats

News flash: treats are not an everyday food. You have to start thinking about healthy food as 'real food' and treats as 'sometimes' foods, or 'junk'. For my weight loss club members, one of the most common reasons for their weight loss slowing down is because they have too many treats, too often, and most of them at the end of the day.

If you want to get real results on the scales every week, leave treats like chocolate, biscuits, cakes or chips (or alcohol if you want to go that far!) off the menu altogether and only use it as an incentive as part of your good week deals. Treat them as a reward for good work done. Get into the habit of savouring how fantastic strawberries and low fat yoghurt tastes, or stone fruits in summer, or Pink Lady apples in winter. Find new foods that you love and eat them when you need a sweet hit, or a crunchy carbohydrate fix.

But if you are going to have a treat (either as a reward or not) make sure you eat it during the day so you can walk some of it off. Never forget that fat is always stored as fat which then has to be worked off your body, and sugar is converted to energy and is only stored as fat when it's not burned off. So eat your treat at lunch or in the afternoon, then go for a long walk. But treats or no treats, stick as much as you can to your calorie and fat intakes for the day.

Incidental exercise

As I said in the chapter on shaking your booty, you need to start exercising in order to shift those kilos. But as well as doing organised or planned exercise at least three times a week, you can also slowly increase your ambient levels of fitness, and burn more calories, by doing more incidental exercise. You can do this really easily by:

- Walking as much as you can everywhere. Don't get in the car for short trips, like the train station or the shops: put your trainers on and walk, baby. Also, get off the train, bus or tram one stop early and walk the rest of the way to your destination.

- Play more outdoor games with your kids; go for weekend family walks together; get a dog and walk it regularly, or walk the neighbour's dog.
- At work, don't take the lift, use the stairs.
- Vigorous house cleaning, gardening, mowing the lawn and car washing can also give you a really good cardio workout.

One of the reasons why Australia has an obesity epidemic is because we have increasingly sedentary lifestyles, so boosting the amount of general physical activity you do, on top of exercising regularly, is going to help keep those kilos falling off as well as give you healthy habits you can use for the rest of your life (not to mention helping our national obesity statistics).

Weekend eating

At the Healthy Body Club I often see food diaries that are perfect during the week but on the weekend everything falls apart – sometimes the amount of food consumed is enough to last three or four days. Socialising always seems to take precedence over exercise, and with a hangover, greasy, post-drinking breakfasts come hand in hand with hours and hours of lying around in bed. Doing a good old-fashioned session of cardio just seems to fall by the wayside.

The other common weekend bust-up (hangover or no hangover) is sleeping in and not eating breakfast till midday, then eating double what you should because by then you are starving. Give yourself a break. Why work so hard during the week to just ruin it all over two days? Give your metabolism a break too. Get up at 9 am and have a drinkable yoghurt on the way to the toilet, *then* go back to bed and sleep till whenever you would normally surface. Keep your metabolism burning. Don't teach it to slow down for two days out of every seven. You are less likely to make a rational decision when you're starving and will probably end up cooking a double serve of bacon, eggs, maple syrup, pancakes and hash browns at mid-morning, then proceed to eat lunch an hour and a half later.

Once again, managing your weekend comes down to planning. During the week, look at your diary and see what you have on. If you are having Saturday lunch in a café with your mates, and Saturday night dinner at a restaurant, then you need to get up early and go to the gym, or go for a power-walk or a run. You could also be having extra 'lean' calorie and fat days on the lead up, and on the other side. Be as honest as you can with yourself about what's going to go into your body over the weekend, including alcohol, and weigh up your options. The bottom line is that you should be making absolutely the best decisions about food until the weekend, and you need to be doing cardio early on the weekends to take the pressure off consuming those extra calories.

It's all about making choices and taking control. If you want to eat out and drink, you have to go easy on the food in the meantime and do some extra work-outs. If you want to take it easy and lay off the exercise over the weekend, then eat lightly and don't drink alcohol.

If you are having brunch, which will be around your mid-morning snack time, get up and have a healthy breakfast – cereal and yoghurt. When you get to the café, have a snack like some raisin toast or a fruit salad or a low fat smoothie. Just because you are at a café doesn't mean you have to eat a main meal because everyone else is. You are not missing out on anything. Food like that will always be there. What do you want more? Bacon and eggs and hash browns at 11 am or that sexy size 12 dress that will slip easily onto your body? You make the choice, because you are in control.

In general, on the weekends make sure you have plenty of fruit in the house. If you are running around doing lots of things then pack a lunch and snacks and avoid having to make a decision about what to eat. It takes five minutes to make a healthy sandwich.

I always find that Sunday night dinners are too hard for me. My soccer game finishes at 5 pm and by the time I get home and have a shower the last thing I feel like doing is cooking. So I prepare for it: I cook a double serve of Friday night's dinner and put one serve in the freezer. On Sunday night, I reheat the leftovers. Easy.

Holiday eating

When I am in holiday-I-know-I-am-going-to-put-on-three-kilos-mode I eat whatever I want but still have certain rules in place, ensuring I make about 60 per cent of my choices the best. This leaves me feeling in control yet happy to have relaxed and enjoyed myself. It's not entirely guilt-free, but that's something I have to continue to deal with and work on for however long it takes me.

For example, if I'm staying in a hotel I will only eat hot food from the breakfast buffet twice in seven days. The rest of the time I have cereal and fruit salad. Also, one of the first things I do is find the local supermarket and stock up on cereal, fruit, bread, low fat ham, licorice, yoghurt and keep it in the bar fridge.

I make sandwiches and take fruit when I am visiting theme parks (I have a small child, remember!) ensuring I can lash out at dinnertime without having to think about the fat-laden burger and fries I haven't had a chance to work off. I could just have a salad for dinner every night (snore) but I want to live my life, and enjoy the food I don't eat very often. The key is to have fun but to also do it in moderation.

Choosing how to eat on your holidays is entirely up to you, though. If you have a deadline for your weight loss, then dropping your 'best' healthy food choice percentage might not be the answer for you at that time. I know, though, that if I have scrimped and saved for a holiday all year, I know I will treat it as just that – a short change in my normal, healthy routine. I make as many good choices as I can, so that still means no thick creamy sauces and no battered fish but on one night I know I *will* eat two kilos of prawns from the all-you-can-eat seafood buffet (and I would like to officially apologise to the Gold Coast Marriott for that!).

Relationship eating

I put on seven kilos in the first year of my previous relationship, then it occurred to me that I could not continue to keep doing it and be happy about it. There was a lot of celebrating, a lot of champagne and chocolates in bed, and too many romantic three-course dinners – eventually I realised the party couldn't go on forever and at some point I had to start making healthy life choices again.

The reality is that a relationship shouldn't make you fat. If you catch yourself saying that your boyfriend makes you fat, you need to remind yourself that you are making the choice to overeat or eat the wrong things, not your boyfriend. Why make excuses like this? Changing the situation may be as simple as making better, healthier choices, being aware of what you are consuming and making time to exercise. You can make a commitment to someone else as well as a healthy life. However, if you're making bad choices because you don't think you have any control or power in the situation, you need to start questioning whether the relationship, or any other things in your life, are as good as they can be. Always actively seek the truth and find solutions, so that you can be as good to yourself as you can be.

That said, I reckon losing weight is much easier when you are single – you are more self-absorbed, you have more time to exercise and you can use the Lean Cuisine method of cooking for one! I think we have all had to sit next to the significant person in our lives gorging their way through a bucket of triple chocolate ice cream. One of the weird things about some blokes is that they just don't care if they put on a few kilos . . . but all this means is that we have to work a little bit harder at making the best choices in these moments, and don't give in to the 'we do everything together, including killing ourselves with crap' way of thinking. You may not be able to get your partner to change, but you can make choices in your own life. You are the mistress of your own destiny. And just how much more chocolate ice cream will he eat when he realises that you are the person being perved on?

If your partner is eating ice cream, and you really feel like some *and* can fit it into your daily tally, then have some low fat ice cream, like Weight Watchers or Dairy Bell. If it's nearly bedtime, have a cup of low fat hot chocolate instead or some lovely herbal tea. When it comes to other food like chocolate or Red Rock Deli chips, being able to say no might be another issue altogether though, so knowing your poison, or knowing what you are most likely to give in to, is the biggest key to keeping a safe house. You are well within your rights to ask that these foods are not brought into the house because it will sabotage something that is very important to you. Explain to your partner that they can eat these things, but just not at home. If your partner loves you and respects the fact that foods like this are forcing you to damage your healthy life choices, they won't have any problem doing this for you. Good relationships rely on fair compromises and doing what it takes to make each other feel safe, healthy and happy.

Schedule social times with your boyfriend, partner or friends outside of your meal-times. For example, instead of meeting friends for breakfast meet them for a walk and have a coffee afterwards. When you have dinner together or with friends, offer to do most of the cooking in return for your partner cleaning up so that the food is more likely to be healthy. If your partner suggests take-away pizza, offer to make it. If you do end up ordering pizza, have one slice and a Lean Cuisine. If you order Thai, get the seafood stir-fry.

If they are receptive, you can help your partner learn about eating and cooking healthily – and if they have some weight to lose themselves, it'll make your own new healthy life so much easier. Don't grow old and fat together. Grow healthy and happy together; you'll live longer!

Now, I'm sure the person who loves you really wants you healthy and happy, but there is a possibility that they might feel better if you stay overweight. A recent study showed that the boyfriends or partners of women who were between size 8 and 12 were more likely to stray than those who had partners a size 14 or above. The findings showed that men with bigger girls were less likely to leave their relationships and/or have an affair.

Why could this be so? Well, for one, the bigger you are the less likely you are to be chatted up or sought after by other men. Sure, there are guys who love big women; I knew many when I was obese, but a lot more men like their women slim, healthy and fit (in other words, these things are attractive to them). If you are being chatted up by a lot more men, your guy may find himself feeling threatened, inadequate and in fear of losing you, so he may encourage you to pile on a few kilos, or sabotage your weight loss plans, in order to feel better about himself.

If you suspect this is going on, he might need reassurance about how much you love him, but also how important losing the weight and getting fit is to you. Perhaps plan romantic getaways as your ongoing weight loss rewards – all he has to do is buy the sexy lingerie – two sizes smaller.

Quick fixes you can use

Here are some great quick fixes of the healthy variety that can help keep you focused when you need it the most.

Quick Fix 1: Make a huge pot of low fat veggie soup. Portion single serves into Tupperware, freeze it, and microwave it for dinner and lunch for a week (eat your snacks as per usual) or for as long as you want it to last. I know someone who'll even eat it for breakfast. It's great for avoiding the decision-making process, particularly when you're feeling vulnerable, like around your period, or when you are stressed at work, which is where a lot of people come off the wagon. You can expect to lose up to a kilo for that week if all your other eating is on track and you are exercising properly. But beware: when you get bored with it (and you will) you are more likely to develop wandering eyes and break out on bad food choices, so make sure you have some other interesting food planned as back-up. In any case, it's better to have a variety of healthy foods and a few treats to keep you motivated.

Quick Fix 2: Do an hour of cardio every day for a week and don't 'eat up'. People who exercise generally eat more because they are hungrier. When you do an hour of hard cardio work (and I don't mean casual walking – I mean running, rowing and sweating) you can get away with consuming another 200 calories in your daily intake. This is the equivalent to two more small snacks a day. If you don't eat these snacks, though, you'll probably see a big difference on the scales for the week.

Quick Fix 3: You go away on holiday and eat, drink and be merry. In a week away you can gain up to four kilos (or is that just me?), depending on how wild you go. Yes, it would be good if you'd eaten healthily and exercised and not drunk fifteen Pina Coladas in the pool bar before going to the Bloody Mary breakfast club, but it's done now and you need to find a solution that will make you happy without putting you on the path to failure.

Have a cooling off period. Don't weigh yourself for the next two weeks and concentrate on the very best healthy eating and lots of exercise. When you do have the weigh-in you may only be a kilo or two heavier, as opposed to the four extra kilos. That small window of time lets you work hard, eat well and atone for your sins. Make this deal with yourself before you go on holidays so you don't feel guilty about having a bit of fun when you're away. You know you have a solution to the holiday weight gain dilemma, so there is a lot less stress involved all round.

Quick Fix 4: For two weeks eat only Lean Cuisines, Weight Watchers meals, or McCain's Healthy Choice frozen meals for dinner. They are fat, calorie and portion controlled and again, prevent you from having to make any decisions. *Always* beef them up with salad or steamed veggies so that you are eating enough and prevent your body going into starvation/famine mode. This is an easy and interesting, albeit slightly more expensive, way to lose that extra kilo. However, I do think that you need to learn to cook because if you have a family, partner, live-in mates or have an active social life, eating these meals continuously just isn't realistic; but in the short term it is OK.

Fine-tune, baby, fine-tune!

- Start fine-tuning to keep getting results
- Eat brekkie! Eat brekkie! Eat brekkie!
- Don't skip meals, you'll only slow down your metabolism
- Control your portions – don't overeat or graze
- Slow down and really relish your meals
- Plan to paint the town red by having lean days before and after and boosting your exercise
- Do more incidental exercise
- Watch your fats and your carbohydrates
- Keep an eye on empty calories like alcohol, sugar and honey
- Eat well on the weekends. Don't go bust
- Don't let anyone stop you from achieving your goals.

Quick Quiz

1. When eating out:
   a) The local all-you-can-eat buffet has a photo of you pinned up, saying 'Under no circumstances serve this person!'
   b) The restaurant cordons off an area so the other customers don't have to see you eat.
   c) You have the degustation menu just for starters.

2. When you go to the movies:
   a) You eat a bucket of popcorn, three choc tops, a jumbo bag of chips and a big bottle of Coke. And that's *before* the movie starts.
   b) You need to book two extra seats – one for your bum, and one for the child you pretended to have so you have somewhere to put all that food.
   c) You get a sore jaw from chewing your way through the entire movie.

3. Christmas is:
   a) A time of giving and joy. You give lots of money to the joyous plastic surgeon who sucks out all the roast pork, ham, mince pies and pudding you ate.
   b) Depressingly filled with too much food and a mother who keeps saying 'Eat, eat!'
   c) When you ask for clothes in a bigger size because by the end of the month you always need them.

Mostly a: You need to read this book.

Mostly b: Please read this book. You really, really need to read this book.

Mostly c: Stop eating this book and read it, please! I mean it!

8

Taking it to the Streets

The lazy girl's survival guide to living real life

'Man cannot discover new oceans until he has the courage to lose sight of the shore.'

Unknown

I think the easiest part of losing weight is eating at home, where you can control your intake and only have the right kinds of foods available when you crave the bad stuff. The hardest part is stepping outside your door – before you know it the world of temptation is in your face, along with all the doughnuts, hot chips and pizza.

You walk past the corner shop and you have to say no to those Kit Kats you used to buy every day. At work there is the skinny girl who always buys Krispy Kreme donuts, not to mention the daily tray of Family Assorted bickies in the kitchen. When you go to lunch you have to survive the food court, the cafe, or the one and only greasy spoon diner that is within walking distance of your work. Then there's the birthday parties, office lunches, after work drinks, girls' nights out, dinner parties, drive throughs, the footy, the beach and the swimming pool – and this is before you start dealing with cravings or the girlfriends who prefer you fatter than they are. Temptation is everywhere.

Unless you are going to live in a bubble for the rest of your life, you have to learn to make good choices with all this temptation swirling around you, despite it being a hell of a lot easier to go to the local drive through and order seventeen meals for you and your invisible friends.

At the Healthy Body Club, where it's imperative to keep a food diary, I often see Oportos, Maccas, KFC, hot chips and pizza where good food choices are supposed to be . . . and along with them, I hear all the same excuses: 'But I ran out of time', 'There was nothing else', 'I was starving and that's where my friends were going'. Now I'm going to be harsh – these excuses are just not good enough to convince me that there was no choice in the situation . . . Hello?! I lost Calista Flockhart off my body! I used those same excuses, too, until the truth of the matter became apparent to me. The truth of the matter was that I was too lazy to be proactive about my own weight loss and healthy life (as well as being downright afraid of reaching my goal).

You have to be prepared. In the beginning, just for a little while, you may just need to avoid situations where there will be temptation until you are strong enough to make decisive, healthy choices in those same situations. But if you do this or not, you should be looking at your diary or calendar for the week ahead anyway so that you know exactly where you are going and what you will be doing. If you know there will be opportunities for temptation (and let's face it, in the furthest reaches of Nepal you can still find a Coke pretty damn easily) you should make and take food with you. Even though I've been doing my healthy eating and living for a few years now I *never* leave the house without my snacks and emergency food. I have a very simple planning exercise: when I'm getting ready to go out I ask myself how long I will be away for, and how many meals I need to take with me

(I even have a sign on the back of my front door to remind me!). I have healthy snacks in the console of my car, and extra snacks in my handbag. I always take fruit and protein bars in case I am out longer than I think. If I am out unexpectedly at a meal time with nothing but bad food choices at my disposal then I can make a temporary healthy choice until I can find something that *is* good for me.

Being prepared like this means that you have to be prepared at home first. You need to have stocks of healthy food like fruit, protein bars, sultana packs or rice crackers in your pantry so they can be grabbed easily and quickly on your way out.

Lunch on the run

When I know I am going to be out over my lunch-time I either make up my own sandwich or a salad first at home, or stop on the way and get a lovely, healthy gourmet sandwich. If I'm going to a picnic I always put together healthy spreads, like salads and fruit platters, that can be contributed to the mix. In these situations, particularly picnics, no-one else ever notices whether you are eating more of one food or the other so just make sure there are good choices on hand and only have small portions of the other stuff.

Managing lunch on the run, again, means that you need to be prepared at home with the right kind of ingredients that can be quickly put together into a quick take-away meal, like bread, lite ham, lite chicken and salad veggies. It also means having the right kind of support gear, like good sandwich bags (the snaplock ones are great because you can re-use them), enough Tupperware or plastic containers you can put sandwiches or salads in, drink bottles for your water, and even a small Esky you can put chilled food into to keep it nice and appetising.

And no time to eat at work, you say? I don't know how busy you are, but you should never compromise your metabolism, or your healthy body pledge to yourself, by not eating. It's just not worth it. You'll work better, and think more clearly, if you eat properly; otherwise you'll get the jitters, lose concentration, start making mistakes, and at 4 pm you won't be able to take it any more and will splurge on some chocolate. If you really must, you can eat at your desk and still keep working, if that's what you have to do – have a cup of low fat instant soup, a high fibre toasted muffin, and some fruit. But as I mentioned in my last chapter, it's important for your body and brain to recognise that you are actually eating a meal, so taking the time to eat slowly and savour your meal is crucial for teaching your body and brain that it has been fed. If you work like this a lot, make sure you have a reliable stash of food that keeps well at work. For example, keep the low fat instant soup in your desk drawer, the high fibre muffins in the freezer in the communal kitchen and some fruit on your desk. Easy.

The movies and the box

I've talked about surviving the movies before in my chapter on emotional eating, and bad habits are the demons that need to be fought off. If you've always snacked on ice cream, chips and lollies when you're seeing a flick, you need to break the habit by taking your own food and creating a new ritual around it. Whenever Kai and I go to the movies, we go straight to the supermarket first and get our air popped, butter free popcorn, baked pretzels, sugar-free Chupa Chups, jelly snakes and two bottles of water. Grapes and strawberries are good, too. Then we watch our film, eating the fantastic food that has cost us about a third of the price, knowing that we have made good food choices that won't catch up with us later. The truth is that, even if you wanted to make a good choice at the candy bar at most cinemas, you couldn't – they sell crap food, they always want to supersize you to boot, as well as take a sizeable chunk out of your wallet. Make a new ritual, instead, of always stocking up on good healthy food that isn't going to kill you in the long run, or murder your bank balance.

Like movie-going, watching the TV can really hinder your weight loss if eating is a habit that goes hand in hand with it. First of all, ask yourself if you are really hungry. If you're watching the box, in all likelihood you've already eaten your dinner, so you're probably *not* hungry. You may just be bored or just feeling the call of the fifteen-year-old bad habit of chewing on something when you're staring slack-jawed at the screen. Don't go there. If you're bored, chances are the program you're watching isn't stimulating, so turn the telly off and do something else on your distraction or nurture list. If telly eating is just an old habit, make something else the new habit, like filing your nails or knitting. Better still, do some sit ups whenever the ads come on. If you are actually hungry, make sure you eat only your post-dinner snack, and make it something healthy like a piece of fruit, some yoghurt, or a low fat hot chocolate drink. If you are going to eat something and be damned, make sure it's not straight from the packet – serve up the right amount, arrange it on a plate, don't go back for seconds, and have a drink of water with it as well.

Social butterfly

If you have a very busy social life and eat out with friends a lot, you may find that hosting dinner parties where you cook all the food is a viable option, instead of blowing precious calories and fat units at the local Thai restaurant. There are plenty of fantastic low fat cookbooks being published now and most people either don't care or won't realise if something is low fat – all they care about is whether it tastes good and there's enough to go around. As well as the obvious benefits of staying in control, it also gives you a great excuse to learn to cook new, healthy and interesting dishes. If there are leftovers, send the single blokes home with a doggie bag, or freeze it for lunches or dinners for the next week.

You may find you start a new trend. The great thing about hosting your own dinner parties is that your friends will invite you over to enjoy their cooking as a return favour. When this happens, call beforehand and let them know you are eating healthily, and ask if they mind you bringing a (healthy) salad to add to the meal. You'll find that most people will either have no problems at all with this, love to have some help with the food preparation, or even accommodate you in their menu. The usually small percentage of people who can't or won't should probably be relegated to the recycled present category of your Christmas list.

If you go to a lot of parties, don't stand next to the table with the nibbles – if food is out of sight, it's out of mind. If you know there's going to be alcohol, always take mineral or soda water with you so you know there is something refreshing and low calorie for you to drink. Also, don't be the first person at the buffet – wait until quite a few people have had a go first, then serve yourself . . . more often than not you'll take a smaller portion because there is less to go around.

If temptation really is a huge problem for you, again, you might need to cut back on your socialising until you feel strong enough to make healthy choices. I'm not telling you to join a nunnery, though – just know your limitations and do whatever it takes to achieve your goals . . . within reason!

Fast food and drive through

Every family in Australia does the drive through or the quick stop-off at the local fast food place (I just can't call it a restaurant, sorry!) – if it's not for yourself then it's to keep the kids from constantly harassing you about the gadget they get, or competition they can enter, with the meal (or just the novelty value of eating somewhere different). Not to mention the convenience factor, of course.

In our house, the rule is that we do it only once a week and only on a day when Kai has exercised, so it's either after swimming or soccer. For me, the hardest part is what I will do when I get there, because I have absolutely zero willpower. The only way for me to manage fast food is either to reduce my access to opportunities where I can make bad choices, or to feed myself beforehand so that I'm not that hungry when we get there. Now, you may be different and be able to order one of the healthier choices at any of the fast food establishments (McDonald's, for example, now has a salads range, a chicken foldover and a healthier hamburger, as well as yoghurt, fruit, cereal and muffins), but I know that if I order the healthy option I *always* follow it up with fries.

So, about three minutes before we arrive, I eat a banana and drink a full bottle of water. It completely fills me up and the thought of eating anything else is actually repellent enough to keep me from ordering anything. The other option, once again, is the sugar-free lollipop. Start sucking it before you get there, and keep sucking it until your child finishes their meal. When you get home, make yourself a healthy sandwich or heat up a quick meal from the freezer, like leftovers or a Lean Cuisine.

If I am out by myself and starving, without a child haranguing me to eat crap food, and there is nothing healthy around at all, I don't give in to the fast food stop-off/drive-through dilemma. Instead I drive to the nearest service station with a mini-market attached, buy a loaf of bread, some lite ham and lite cheese, and throw together a very quick and relatively healthy sandwich. If the range is really limited, I grab a banana or a protein shake from the fridge, or a yoghurt or low fat muesli bar. There really is no excuse for eating food that is bad for you and your goals. If you find yourself at the local fast food establishment it's because you want to eat the food, not because it was the only choice available to you. Remember, wherever there is a fast food joint, there is always a service station just a bit further down the road.

Stay focused, be prepared and honour your body. You will be amazed at how good you feel once you have learned to take control. Making healthy choices is much more satisfying than oil-soaked fries. I promise.

Drinking

When I am in weight-loss mode I always cut my alcohol intake down to a minimum. I don't cut it out completely because prohibition doesn't work. The more something is unavailable, the more desirable it becomes. But despite all the current recommendations about healthy adults being able to have up to two glasses of wine per night, I see those two glasses only as extra calories that I don't need.

Now, I am no saint. I have been known to consume twenty-seven beers in one night and still be able to mutter my name. It does sound a bit like I'm trying to speak Japanese, and yes, on one occasion I did break my leg, but the point I am making is that I like a drink or two . . . hundred. It's not easy giving it up. But it's also not easy seeing another summer slip by, avoiding the beach because you can't stand the thought of the water jumping out when you jump in. It's about having priorities and reducing the temptation of having another drink, and then another, and then another and then . . . well, you get the idea.

I save my drinking for special occasions – and I mean *really* special. Not just the opening of an envelope, which can seem pretty spectacular after weeks of lemon, lime and sodas. There are a few things I do to minimise my alcohol intake, at home and at play. There is a handy section in the previous chapter on finetuning, on keeping limits in place when you are drinking, but here are some extra ideas on actually cutting back without anyone noticing (including yourself, sometimes!):

AJ's alcohol busters

1. After a long day, I would always have a glass of wine in the bath at night. Now, I do everything in exactly the same way – candles, music, incense and bath bombs, but I have apple juice in a wine glass instead. It looks and tastes like wine, and is still sweet, but it doesn't make me want to drink more, and then subsequently eat more with the alcohol munchies.
2. When I've cooked my yummy, healthy meal, I put water in a wine glass, dim the light so that it's not so apparent to me the water is not wine, and settle in for a relaxed dinner.

3. If I am out, I have a two-drink rule, which becomes a three-drink rule if I am out very late. When I arrive, I have my first drink, which is generally vodka and soda in a tall glass. The social comfort and ice breaking factors are taken care of with that one, first drink. Then I drink soda in a tall glass, with the added bonus of nobody noticing that I don't have alcohol in my glass. Half-way through the night I have my next vodka and soda in a tall glass. If I am out dancing till the wee hours, I may have another but generally don't really want it because I can see just how drunk everyone else is. This system works really well because no-one realises you're not drinking as much as them; there's minimum peer group pressure and you can even trick yourself by having the same glass and mixer (I often forget that I'm not actually drinking alcohol). I also drink soda and diet lime in a tumbler with ice cubes if I really want to have the taste of something in my mouth.

4. If I'm at a dinner party, I always take mineral or soda water with me so that I know there is something for me to drink that isn't alcohol; and sometimes will hang the expense and buy a really lovely bottle of wine, which I can share around and savour slowly (with one or two glasses only) throughout the meal. If it's a really good bottle of wine, it'll be so popular that there'll only be one or two glasses to drink anyway!

5. Most cocktail bars have one or two alcohol-free drinks, like Virgin Marys (a Bloody Mary without the vodka), which can give me the extravagant feeling of a cocktail but with none of the consequences.

6. If I really need to keep my mouth or hands busy when I'm out, sugar-free lollipops or chewing gum can do just as good a job as another glass of alcohol (and an even better job than smoking – yuck!).

7. I always have an ever-present bottle of water with me in my bag, or in my hand (especially at parties which stops me from reaching for the nibblies as well).

8. Don't get caught up in rounds of shouts. You'll feel

compelled to drink more to keep up and get your money's worth. Tell people you're in training for a fun run (never tell people you're dieting!) and that you're skipping the rounds.

9. Don't keep wine or beer in the fridge – it's too much of a temptation in your moments of weakness.

10. Last, but never least – don't drink on an empty stomach!

I know these things may sound a bit ridiculous but drinking, particularly when you are out with your friends, is a habit that can be broken. You don't actually have to be pissed to have a good time; people appreciate you for who you are, not for what alcohol does to you. Sometimes, simply replicating the experience of a glass of wine or a cocktail is enough to make you feel as though you aren't missing out. Of course, if your circle of friends are alcoholics and the only time you ever see them is when they are drunk, this may become a bit boring for you if you are committed to cutting back on the alcohol. You might want to find some new friends.

Eating out

OK, this is the meaty bit. Eating out can be the killer of any weight loss goal. If you are anything like me, you have to be strong and be prepared.

The golden rule is: never go out to dinner when you are hungry. I know that sounds stupid, but let me explain. As soon as you enter the 'Oh my god, I'm so hungry I could eat a horse' zone, you are in trouble. You've done your dash before you've even started eating. How many times have you been so hungry that you end up eating twice as much as you'd planned, and four times more than you needed? Remember, food is fuel. Any more than that is called comfort eating.

Before you go out to eat anywhere, remind yourself of your weight loss goal. Try on your skinny jeans, read your pledge and think of the body that you want. Acknowledge that food will always be there; you don't have to eat everything in sight, you are not missing out. You are gaining a whole new body and lease on life.

Then eat something healthy before you leave. Before going out to dinner I have a small snack – a banana, a smoothie or a protein bar. These things keep my hunger at bay and help me to make a healthier choice. You are so much less likely to make a rational, healthy decision about food if you are driven by rapacious hunger. Then the panic sets in, and you feel anxious that you won't eat enough to satisfy your hunger . . . and you choose comfort food, and big servings of it as well.

Make sure you enjoy yourself but don't overindulge, and don't let others convince you to have more than you need. Remind them that you really want to be healthy and you would appreciate it if they supported you in achieving your goals. If all else fails change the subject. There's nothing like a bit of ranting and raving about religion and politics to take the emphasis away from what you're eating. Whatever works for you.

Now let's look at what you can eat. The real key is

Here are my golden rules for eating out:

1. If you are going out, make sure you do a cardio work-out the day before, the day in question and the day after. No excuses. You should also have 'lean' eating days before and after.
2. As I mentioned, eat a healthy snack before you go out to stave off ravenous beast behaviour.

3. Stay away from the bread, herb bread, and garlic bread. If the wait-staff put complimentary bread on your table, ask them to take it away.

4. Drink water while waiting for your meal, and sip it throughout the meal.

5. Do not eat three courses. Save that for your celebration meal for when you hit your goal weight (although you probably won't feel like it then).

6. If you must eat two courses, one has to be a totally healthy choice (for example, fruit salad without the ice cream, salad with dressing on the side, plain oysters etc). If you do want two courses, ask for both to be served at entrée sizes. Otherwise, choose one entrée-sized meal, and have a glass of wine.

7. Cheat the dessert course by having a taste of your partner's or friend's.

8. Control how your meal is served. If something is served with fries, don't trust yourself to leave them on your plate, ask for the meal without them. Also, be proactive about how your meal will be cooked – ask if the fish is grilled with oil, and veto the oil if it is. Always ask for sauces and dressings on the side so it is *your* decision how much to use on your meal, not the gluttonous chef's.

9. Unless all meals are served in small portions (like in fancy restaurants, where the more you pay means the less you get), never eat all that you are served. Restaurants do not serve up healthy portions – for example, they overdo it with gargantuan pieces of meat that would keep Godzilla going for a week, and serve it upon enormously-sized plates that make the meal look normal-sized. Keep a mental picture or idea of the size of the meal you should be eating and stick to it on the plate (remember your 'four quarters' portion sizing). If you are able to serve yourself, this makes things a bit easier.

10. Eat slowly. It takes twenty minutes for your body to recognise it is full. Take your time and listen to your body.

choosing a restaurant with healthy possibilities. Obviously, German restaurants and fast food outlets are a bit limited in terms of their menus, but the good news is that, at most restaurants, there will generally always be something you can eat without spoiling all your hard work. As a general rule, any food that has been stir-fried, steamed, grilled, poached or baked will probably be OK, but you never know where those evil chefs are injecting their lard or beef tallow, so always ask questions about the meal you're thinking of ordering. Avoid anything you think is probably fried or battered, cooked in oil or butter, is creamy with sour cream, cream or coconut milk, or crumbed. If you're ordering sandwiches or focaccia, always ask for no butter or margarine, ask for any salad dressing to come on the side, and ask for no added salt. At the end of the day, it's about using your common sense – if the food isn't something you'd eat or cook at home, don't choose it when you're at a restaurant.

Japanese
Healthy choice: Any clear, stock-based soup (e.g. miso), udon noodle soup, steamed dumplings, steamed or stir fried veggies, braised or grilled chicken, beef and fish, tofu, steamed rice, chicken teriyaki, pickled veggies, sashimi, sushi rolls, california rolls, nori rolls.

Avoid: Any fried food (tofu, chicken, seafood or veggies), tempura, Gyoza, chicken or pork katsu, teppanyaki.

Spanish
Healthy choice: Ensalda mixta (salad), pulpo a la vinagreta (octopus vinaigrette), mejillones con aguacate (mussels), sopa de ajo (garlic soup), alcachofas salteadas (sautéed artichoke hearts), gambas al ajillo (garlic prawns), trucha al tinto (trout in red wine sauce), langostinos a la plancha

(grilled prawns), pollo al ajillo (garlic chicken), chipirones rellenos (stuffed squid). Stick to seafood, chicken and salads; anything grilled is good, the red wine sauce and veggies in vinaigrettes are also good choices.

Avoid: Queso de cabra montañes (baked goat cheese), buñuelos de verdure (cauliflower, broccoli cheese puffs), gambas con gabardina (butter fried prawns), vieiras al azafrán (scallops in cream), croquetas de pollo (chicken croquettes), pato braseado (roast duckling), lomito al cabrales (pork with goat cheese), butifarras con brevas (pork sausage), chorizo a la plancha (grilled spanish sausage), queso rebozado con miel (fried cheese). Steer clear of any deep fried or fried food, as well as any sausages (e.g. chorizo), ham, creamy sauces and cheese (I know you hate me).

Thai

Healthy choice: Fresh rice paper rolls with veggies, BBQ octopus, clear soups like tom yum goong, tom jued, po tak, wonton soup etc, yum nua (salad), beef salad, stir fries with chicken, vegetables or seafood, Thai chilli sauce, soy and oyster sauce, garlic prawns, pad talay (prawns, fish, calamari, mussels, shallots and basil), pad pak goong (veggies in oyster sauce), any steamed or stir fried seafood dishes, steamed rice.

Avoid: Deep fried spring rolls, curry puffs, fried calamari, money bags or dim sims, satay (peanut) sauce, fish cakes, anything cooked in or with coconut milk, for example tom kha gai, goong choo chee, tom kha pak or laksa, massaman curry, green or red curry, omelette, fried rice.

Chinese

Healthy choice: Wonton soup, any clear stock-based noodle soup, steamed dumplings and dim sims, steamed veggies, steamed or stir fried chicken, beef or seafood with veggies (like chicken chop suey, and chow mein beef, chicken pork or seafood), steamed rice, tofu with vegetables, garlic prawns, sweet and sour prawns.

Avoid: Spare ribs, egg drop soup, fried dumplings, deep fried spring rolls and dim sims, fried rice, crispy noodles, duck, prawn toast, sweet and sour pork, lemon chicken, pork in plum sauce.

Italian

Healthy choice: Marinated calamari, steamed mussels, garlic prawns, garlic calimari, any dish or pasta with a tomato sauce base, marinara sauce, baked or grilled fish, veal or chicken marsala, thin crust pizza with vegetable toppings, minestrone, gelato (made with ice, not cream).

Avoid: Any kind of stuffed vegetable, like artichokes and mushrooms, fried calamari, cheesy meat-filled pasta, for example lasagne, tortellini, cannelloni or ravioli, gnocci, alfredo sauce, pesto, meat sauce, carbonara sauce, pancetta, veal, chicken or eggplant parmesan, thick crust pizza with meaty or cheesy toppings, garlic bread, herb bread, tiramisu, gelato (cream based).

French

Healthy choice: Salade niçoise, steamed mussels, meat, fish or chicken with wine-based sauces, consommé, anything 'la provençale' or tomato-based, bouillabaisse, ratatouille, steamed veggies, seafood soups, dips like tapenade, rouille.

Avoid: Fondue, crepes, croissants, brioche, any soup with cream, pâté de foie gras, anything stuffed, anything 'au gratin', béarnaise, béchamel, hollandaise, veloute or mornay sauces, soufflé, fondue, kidneys, duck, liver.

General
Healthy choice: Green salad, hamburger (plain only), salad sandwich, roast beef sandwich, chicken breast sandwiches, tuna and salmon sandwiches, ham and salad sandwiches, baked potato, grilled fish, chicken breast salad, pancakes (no butter), poached eggs, fruit toast with jam only, egg white omelette, skim milk smoothies, fruit compote, bagels.

Avoid: Fries, chips, or wedges, burgers with bacon, egg and cheese, or burgers 'with the lot', fish burgers, fried chicken, schnitzel, chicken nuggets, deep fried chicken, egg sandwiches, fried eggs, sausages, sausage sandwiches, croissants, risotto, caesar and greek salads, fried fish, ribs.

Easter and Christmas (or anything that involves Jesus)

The reason why Jesus and God are so big at Easter and Christmas is because it's the first thing you say when you step on the scales a week after the event!

Easter
Easter is simultaneously a time of great celebration and great depression. The merchandise hits the shops early (only a few weeks after Christmas), ads for the chocky bunnies and eggs are on every minute of the day and everybody you know – and even some you don't – buy you chocolate. I know, I know. You can stop screaming now, I've stopped.

Once again, you can't make the world free of temptation but there are things you can do to avoid a complete burnout. The phrase, as always, is be prepared. Or, in the case of Easter, don't give in to it.

Tell your close family and loved ones that you are not eating chocolate this year (you have discovered a dormant allergy to cocoa, or that you are lactose intolerant, whatever it takes) and that you would prefer them to give you an instant lottery ticket instead. You could also encourage them to give the money or the chocolate to a charity of your choice. Some people, determined to sabotage your efforts (a topic I will cover later in this chapter), will ignore you. This is where you have to be strong. Remember that it is *only* chocolate. There will always be chocolate. The world is full of it. It's not going to run out. You are not on death row; it is not your last meal. You will be able to eat chocky again, but just not now. And finally, always remember that the body you want will not happen unless you make healthy choices.

If you do end up with a generous stash of eggs and chocolates *do not leave them in the fridge or pantry* for that magical day when you will be able to have it. Don't presume you will be strong enough to ration them out. Willpower doesn't exist. You have to make your house safe. Having chocolate in the fridge doesn't make your house safe. If you are seriously overweight, Easter temptation in the form of chocolate and hot cross buns is sure to be one of your major downfalls so make it easy for yourself and get rid of it. Think about it – it's not just the Easter weekend that accounts for retailers' huge profits in chocolate and doughy buns, it starts two months before and finishes a month later. That's a potential three months' worth of temptation and bad choices. You can undo all your good work in three months. Don't let it happen.

Of course, though, getting and staying healthy in the lazy girl way is not about prohibition – it's about portion control and allowable treats. Allow yourself two small eggs to eat as part of a good week deal and then bundle the rest up and palm them off on whoever will take them. Last year I sent them to vacation care with Kai and he was the most popular kid there. The year before that I lived around the corner from an aged and handicapped persons' home. They were very grateful for my generous gift of unopened chocolate. When I was in hospital with my broken leg I received three boxes of chocolates (interestingly, from people who knew I was trying to lose weight). I gave those boxes of chockies to the nurses, which meant that I got painkillers whenever I wanted. There are plenty of people who would love the extra chocolate – kindergartens, the postman, the garbos, the workers at your local homeless shelter (whoever thanks them?). And remember, when you give, people give back in other ways.

Palm off the chocolate as soon as you get it. If someone at work puts an egg on your desk, pick it up and give it to the mail boy. The longer it is in your possession the more likely you are to succumb to temptation. Chocolate (on this scale) is the instrument of the devil! It must be exorcised from your life, otherwise it will have to be exercised from your hips. Which would you prefer?

What to do when craving chocolate

1. Try on that pair of jeans that used to fit you (weren't the eighties great? Luckily most of those fashions are coming back). Cringe. Palm off the chocky.
2. Find a brightly-lit change room and force your cottage cheese bum and legs into a size 10 bikini. Scrutinise closely. Cringe. Go home, palm off the chocky.
3. Go to local liposuction clinic for an appraisal. After five minutes with the size 6 assistant, Tiffany, you'll be back at the gym for a five-hour workout before snacking on lettuce leaves for the next ten years. Again, go home, palm off the chocky.

Now, knowing there is going to be lots of chocolate doing the rounds at this time of year, it is reasonable to assume that you will probably crave it even more than usual. Make it easier on yourself and have allowable chocolate treats in your house. Stock up on lots of diet chocolate mousse, low fat fudge brownies and chocolate protein bars for those cravings you just can't ignore.

Christmas

If your family is anything like mine there was always enough food on the table to feed a small nation all day, every day for the entire twelve days of Christmas . . . and then some. But there is no need for you to have a setback at this time of year. With a little extra effort you are sure to have a happy Christmas with food that tastes great without putting those extra kilos on. You know I am going to say it again, so here goes . . . the key is *being prepared*!

There are lots of things you can do to make this time a lot easier on yourself. Hopefully you've told your family what you are doing and they eagerly support you in your quest for a healthy body. First of all, offer to host the family feast at your place. You can cook up a healthy three course meal that everyone can enjoy, and all you have to do is control your portions and your alcohol. Most slimming magazines have great recipe ideas a few months before the big day (or days) so save them up and pull them out when you need them.

If someone else insists on hosting the get-together, offer to cook something to contribute to the menu. Perhaps encourage the family to go on a picnic instead where everyone brings something (and you take healthy, lite ham, turkey, prawns or oysters and a salad). Seafood is really popular at this time of year, and it's healthy, so it's a great choice to have around.

When you're shopping for the big family feasts, buy all the treat food, for example peanuts, Christmas cake, chips, etc, just a few days before the big day; better still, on Christmas Eve. If these things sit around your house for weeks before the main event you'll be tempted to crack them open and have just a few, and before you know it you are back in the supermarket buying it all again. Keep a safe house at all times.

On the big day, nibblies can bring your healthy eating plan undone from the get go. Take healthy alternatives wherever you go, like baked pretzels, air popped popcorn or rice crackers. Don't stand near the nibblies table, and keep your own healthy stash near you. Before you sit down to the main meal, have a banana and drink some water so you don't consume enough food to feed the entire English army. *Always* have water on hand; it'll reduce your alcohol intake and make sure you don't overeat from dehydration. If you are attending a big meal in the evening then make an extra healthy choice during the day by just eating salad or a Lean Cuisine.

After the big meal, don't go lolling around on all the available furniture (you won't feel like it anyway, because you haven't stuffed yourself to high heaven). Encourage everyone to get out and go for a family walk, or a swim in the pool, or a game of soccer. It'll burn off at least some of the food you have eaten.

Just because there's lots of great food around at this time of year does not mean you have to eat only carrot sticks and alfalfa sprouts. For every fattening choice there is an equally satisfying non-fattening choice. You just have to look around for the things that work for you. As I mentioned earlier, every year in the lead up to Christmas every slimming magazine will have a Christmas special with lots and lots of fantastic low fat, calorie controlled ideas about what to cook and eat – everything from full three course meals to low fat

Low fat alternatives

Christmas cake: low fat fudge brownies (Betty Crocker is my fave)

Ham off the bone: shaved light honey cured ham

Roast chicken: a few slices of chicken breast with no skin (remember, chicken skin is full of saturated fat!)

Roast turkey: a few slices of turkey breast with no skin

Roast veggies: veggies oven baked in foil

Gravy: there are stacks of low fat gravies at the supermarket these days

Trifle: diet jelly, peaches and low fat custard

Chips/nuts: baked pretzels (e.g. Parkers), Chinese rice cracker mixes

Crackers and dip: low fat seaweed rice crackers and low fat dip (Weight Watchers have a good range)

Lollies: sugar-free Chupa Chups, red licorice, jelly snakes

Alcohol: water, soda water, mineral water, any 'diet' sodas or cordials, wine spritzers.

treats you can have when everyone else is tucking into the festive nuts.

Birthdays and rewards

So many of my Healthy Body clubbers absolutely dread their birthdays because of all the temptation that comes with it; or they have a great birthday but spend the rest of the week partying hard and then give up on their weight loss efforts because they feel as if they have failed.

One of the most common excuses I hear is about birthday cakes: 'But they made it especially for me.' Just because someone makes something for you doesn't mean you have to eat it . . . all! You can also accept the cake with your best smile, thank them, have a small slice, and then give the rest of the cake to someone else who will appreciate it. Remember – it's your birthday, and you can do whatever *you* want to do. If your skinny friend really wants to go to a German restaurant, all expenses paid, let them go – alone. There are plenty of other things you can ask for, or hint at, instead of going to an upmarket restaurant. Have a look at the list on page 206. If someone offers you a drink and you don't want it, don't drink it. (If someone hands you a drink and says 'This will make your thighs expand to twice their size', would you drink it? No. I've made my point.) If anyone insists you snack on sausages when you are trying to lose weight, chances are this person is not good for you and should be scratched off your Christmas card list. Be strong. Visualise what you want and stick to the limits you have set yourself.

It is actually OK to have a small slice of cake and have a few drinks, but if you are going out to eat, choose somewhere that has healthy choices. You may even want to host your own dinner party and control the food that way. Make your own healthy low fat birthday cake (there are hundreds of fab cake recipes in magazines, on the net, in cookbooks) – I cook a hell of a low fat tiramisu (see page 317).

It's one thing to wake up on your birthday feeling dissatisfied with your body, but it's a completely different thing not to do anything about it. Be proactive – empower yourself. Think of the next birthday and that great dress you will fit into and that extra cake or champagne won't seem so attractive after all.

Similarly, don't congratulate yourself with food. We often celebrate life achievements by eating certain things, or in a certain way, and end up with 'happy' foods (for me it was Pluto Pups at the Easter show) that sabotage our weight loss.

When we graduate from school, college or university we celebrate by eating out at a ritzy restaurant. We celebrate motherhood with chocolates and champagne, and sporting achievements with four-course dinners and unlimited alcohol. This has to change – there are always going to be life achievements like this. Instead of going to a restaurant, ask your family and friends to contribute to a holiday fund (you can arrange this at any travel agency; they'll give you special 'hand out' cards with the booking number on it).

Write a long list of alternative rewards or achievement celebration gifts. I have mine written down at home and often remind friends and family that these are things I would like instead of being wined and dined. You can also use these for your weight loss goal rewards, too. Here are mine:

AJ's achievement rewards

Write yours:

Versace Woman (perfume) _____

Skydiving vouchers _____

Horse riding vouchers _____

Manicures and pedicures _____

New clothes _____

Jewellery _____

Massages _____

Weekends away _____

Theatre tickets _____

Pushers and saboteurs

These people come in all shapes and sizes, however they are generally thinner, younger and fitter than you. They can be disguised as doting grandmothers, insistent mothers, friendly co-workers, generous friends or gracious hostesses who have 'slaved all day to make it, now have some more!'

I don't know why some people are like this, but I have more than a few in my life. They can be friends and colleagues who don't understand why you want to change, or don't want to acknowledge that you are in the process of changing your body and your life for the better. Generally pushers and sabo-teurs are feeling threatened by your new sense of control and focus, may want to keep you right where you are because it's safe for them (they may be just that little bit thinner than you and have thus always considered themselves 'better' than you), simply can't grasp what you are doing because they have their own convoluted eating or weight issues, or have always been thin and have never had to lose weight. Some people love to control others by feeding them; others feel that the only way they know how to nurture is with food. If you have friends who are overweight as well, the attention you get because you are losing weight might make them feel insecure, unsafe or jealous. Parents in particular might feel more comfortable if you are overweight – you don't go out as much, and you have more time to spend with them.

You need to learn to say no to people like this, and some people will insist until they are blue in the face (I lost a friendship with the person who always brought junk around to my house, despite my constant protestations). Personally I like to deal with some people by pulling up my shirt, and talking to my belly in a baby voice just as the pusher hostess walks by: 'Does jelly belly want any more crackers, cheese and dippy wippy? I don't think so!' If that doesn't work I start knocking expensive ornaments off the shelves with my bum and exclaim loudly 'Whoa, any more meatballs and the walls will go down. Bring those nibblies in here, Maureen.'

But seriously, there are a number of things you can do to help yourself:

1. When people offer you their treats, nibblies or second helpings, politely refuse. If someone insists, then use the technique developed by Allen Pease, who wrote a book called *Talk Language*. It is called 'broken record' language. You say the same thing over and over again without giving them any more information – for example, say 'Thanks but no thanks' and nothing else. If you give people more information like 'I'm trying to lose weight' you are giving them ammunition to argue their point with. They can say things like 'You don't need to lose weight, you look fine. Have some dip.' The less ammunition you give them, the less they have to argue with. By the time you have repeated the same thing three times in a row they will give up and move on to annoy someone else (that is, unless they are completely insane).

2. If the person seems reasonable and is a good friend, take them aside and explain your situation and enlist their help. People love to be asked for help, especially if control is one of their personality traits. If they feel like spoiling you, ask them to buy you fruit, a scratch lottery ticket, or anything else on your alternative rewards list.

3. If any food pushing happens at dinner with friends or family, change the subject, offer to help clear the table or serve dessert (which will also enable you to discreetly alter your portion size).

4. If a pusher ignores you and puts food in front of you (like on your desk at work) saying 'I'll just leave it here in case you change your mind' give it straight back and say, 'I said "no thanks".' Or give it to someone else immediately, or simply throw it in the bin, preferably if they are still watching. If they insist again, just say 'I said "no thanks".'

Remember, you are responsible for making *yourself* happy – as soon as you start thinking about what others want or need, you immediately put your own priorities aside. If your mum insists you eat some cheesecake, be strong – you don't want the cheesecake, you don't need the cheesecake. Tell her you love her and while you're giving her a hug tell her that you'd really just prefer some fruit.

Prepare for the 'worst'

Losing weight successfully is not about that elusive Oprah-like willpower we imagine everyone else has. The reality is that Oprah is just like everyone else. She had to work really hard to lose a large amount of weight. There are some things you can do to make it easier on you so that it's not so much hard work, though. Knowing *when* you give in to temptation and snack, graze and comfort eat is a very powerful tool in breaking bad habits.

This is where your food diary comes in handy – not just on a daily or weekly basis, but monthly as well. Analyse your food diary and see if you can spot a pattern where you eat extra calories or where you have your crashes and burns. If you do find a pattern, great! It's fixable; there are lots of solutions to all kinds of problem times. You might find an over-eating pattern in the late afternoon or at night, watching TV, or a weekly mini blow-out every Friday evening at the office drinks session.

For example, take going to the footy. What do people do at the footy? Drink beer and eat pies. You may be justifying it by saying that 'I *have* to have a meat pie at the footy. That's what I always do'. But think about this: you might *always* struggle to fit into a size 12 pair of jeans just because you have two pies and three beers at the footy. I understand completely why we do this. It's a tradition. For some of my friends, it's a family tradition they have been doing since they were four years old, and it is an Australian tradition. Meat pies are pretty much synonymous with the football.

But Australia is also synonymous with obesity – we have one of the highest rates of obesity in the world! Just because you've always done something doesn't mean it is right, and it doesn't mean you have to keep doing it. It certainly doesn't mean you won't have fun if you don't eat pies and drink beer.

If you find something like this in your food diary, recognise that the food you are eating has become tangled up with the experience of doing something else that is fun (it has become a 'happy' food). You need to reprogram yourself with a new, healthy 'happy' food – if you're going to the footy, make a fantastic picnic hamper with similar, but healthy, food. For example, low fat frittata, if it's cooked in deep pie trays, looks and tastes as good as a pie, and diet ginger ale can look and taste as good as a beer.

Another common pattern time may be eating pub grub on a Friday night. It might be at the pub, or it might be being replicated at home – steak, chips, deep fried fish and cala-mari – Fridays are traditional end of the week let-downs for a lot of people, and families. Recognise it as a pattern that is undoing your weight loss, and make a new, special ritual of the Friday night meal. Pore over your recipe books during the week and and decide on the 'special' meal. Shop and prepare all the food, so that when you and your partner are ready to eat, it's easy to cook (even for him!). Arrange every-thing like a cooking show, and show off the prawns that are shelled, with the ingredients chopped and measured out in small stainless steel bowls. You'll have an evening meal that is freshly cooked, low fat and delicious as well as being a 'special' Friday night feed. If you have kids, involve them in the making of the dinner – if they're old enough, they can decide which special meal they'd like to eat, and help with the cooking.

Go through your food diary for the last month and note all the patterns you can see where you overeat or eat the wrong kind of food. For example:

- Fridays – work lunch
- Once a month it is somebody's birthday at work, or morning tea – cake
- Friday night – boyfriend always orders pizza
- Saturday morning breakfast – café
- Every early evening preparing dinner for the kids – grazing on their food

Once you have identified where you come unstuck, create an action plan to avoid crashing and burning at personal, social and professional events. For example:

Friday – work lunch
Ring the restaurant or pub you are going to. Ask them to fax the menu to you beforehand so you know what you are going to eat, without having to make a decision at the restaurant under pressure. Perhaps even order your meal before you go so you don't have to make a decision at all when you are there. If there are no healthy choices, suggest another venue with a broader range and some healthy choices.

Birthdays and morning teas at work
This is a very common problem. Some workplaces actually have a fund that pays for the food at these get-togethers.

First of all you can offer to make a cake with some money from the cake fund, so you can control what is going into your mouth (and everyone else's). You can also eat beforehand, like some yoghurt, or something else that is protein-based and substantial (and thus low GI) so it will keep your hunger at bay. If you eat beforehand it really controls that internal argument you have over whether to eat the cake or not: if you're not hungry, you can have a small piece if you really want some, then only eat half of it and discretely dispose of the rest (preferably not into the pot plant!) – no fuss made. You can also make some suggestions to the person organising the morning tea or celebration, like buying fruit as well as cakes and biscuits, or low fat dips and rice crackers. You could even go as far as mentioning 'occupational health and safety' at some point. See how quickly some bananas and apples turn up at the next do!

Friday night – boyfriend always orders pizza
Your bloke or partner has probably done this since they were single and sharing a house with people who couldn't, or wouldn't, cook. Recognise this as their bad habit and don't allow it to become yours. Have the ingredients to make your own pizzas and do that instead. If all else fails, have one slice of pizza and then eat a Lean Cuisine. Something to keep in mind, though, is that most slices of pizza average about 20 grams of fat – half your daily intake!

Saturday morning breakfast – café
Instead of going to the café, go for an early morning walk and pick up some fresh bread rolls. Poach eggs and grill some low fat bacon and have a yummy, healthy breakfast at home. Set up a table in the backyard, turn on some music, get out the newspapers and recreate a café atmosphere.

Every late afternoon – preparing dinner for the kids

Make sure you have lots of fruit and chilled water on hand when you're making the little tacker's meal so you don't eat their leftovers. Make sure you have a double snack in the afternoon so you aren't hungry, or have a low fat hot chocolate drink while you are cooking and cleaning up. Remember, leftovers should go in the bin only (and you're not a bin, so why treat yourself like one?). Only cook your kids healthy food (they have a right to be healthy, too), so that if you do have a little, it won't hurt so much.

Now, write your list, approach each one separately and make a safer life for yourself and your goals.

Times I struggle to make healthy choices

_____

_____

_____

_____

_____

_____

_____

_____

Don't let lack of preparation lead you to temptation

Life goes on and there will always be challenges like food temptations, risky environments and pushers. Locking yourself up is not the answer, though. It might be good to do it for a little while if you know you need to bolster your decision-making skills, but in the long run you need to be out there, dealing with life as it comes to you. Learning to be strong and prepared is important in creating a safe and healthy environment that supports your weight loss, health and fitness goals.

A healthy life is not about going without. It's about knowing when to treat yourself and when to make healthy choices. It's also about learning to treat yourself with healthy choices, rather than with food that sets you back and ultimately makes you feel bad about yourself. Just get on with living a healthy life, pick yourself up when you fall over, and keep going until you fall over again. As long as you keep getting up, nothing will get in the way of you achieving your goals – no matter how long it takes. It's not a race. You will get there when you are ready. It's better to get there eventually than to give up because you haven't done it within a certain time frame and 'failed'.

Just one last word on doing what it takes to achieve your dreams. I know it can seem hard making so much of an effort to constantly be prepared, to take food with you, to find the low fat alternatives. But that's not hard. *Hard* is trying to squeeze a size 26 bum into size 12 jeans. *Hard* is trying to fit your obese body into an airline seat without the person sitting next to you requesting they sit in the baggage compartment instead. *Hard* is trying to love yourself when you are stuffing fifteen slices of pizza down your throat. If you genuinely want to be healthier, fitter and happier then do what it takes to get your eating under control. All you have to do is take five minutes out of the day to make a sandwich, thirty minutes to go for a run or a walk, and a few minutes each week to plan what's coming up in your life so that you, other people and life in general doesn't sabotage your weight loss. It's really not as hard as you think.

Survive real life

- Be prepared
- Never leave home without thinking about where you are going or for how long you will be gone
- Take food with you: picnics, parties, dinners, snacks – whatever it takes to stick to your goals
- Stock up your handbag, car, workplace and kitchen with emergency rations
- Rearrange your social life to be centred around activity rather than food
- Cut down your alcohol intake by drinking spritzers, low cal drinks or water instead
- Always have water on hand (carry a water bottle wherever you go)
- Keep busy to avoid unnecessary grazing
- Work out on heavier food days
- Always keep a safe house. Don't hold on to food that you don't need (chocolate, lollies, cooking oil, butter)
- Be proactive. Find foods that are similar to the ones you crave
- Once you've cleaned out your cupboard, clean out your closet of friends – anyone who doesn't support you, goes
- Use your food diary to tell you when you are coming unstuck. Be proactive about finding solutions
- Be prepared.

Quick Quiz

1. When the going gets tough:
   - a) You get going to the nearest fast food take-away outlet.
   - b) You eat until you feel sick, then you eat more because you feel terrible that you ate so much.
   - c) You eat some carrot sticks and sesame seeds and meditate until your troubles melt away.

2. When you hit a weight loss plateau:
   - a) You eat your way to a ten-kilo weight gain so you don't have to think about reaching your goal weight.
   - b) You starve yourself till you crack the plateau, then binge your way back over it, then starve your way back under it again.
   - c) You relax. When it happens it will be the perfect time for it to happen.

3. 'Plateau' means:
   - a) Pathetically Large Arse Too Enormous And Ugly.
   - b) That you were never meant to be a size 10 – just a 14 and then a 16 and then an 18 . . .
   - c) A time to really push yourself. You enjoy the challenge your body presents you.

Mostly a: You really should have shares in KFC and Burger King. Please stop eating for five minutes and read this chapter . . . but wipe the grease off your fingers first.

Mostly b: I have one word for you: yo-yo. Actually, that's two words, not counting the hyphen. If you want to learn how to crack the damn plateau sensibly, read this chapter.

Mostly c: Listen here, Moonbeam River Dance Moccasin Pussybush the third, some of us have consumed entire cows – and yes, we did enjoy it. Go deep-fry some alfalfa sprouts . . . you might understand where we're coming from!

9

Get Off the Dreaded Plateau

'You will have wonderful surges forward. Then there must be a time
of consolidation before the next forward surge. Accept this as part of
the process and never become downhearted.'

Eileen Caddy, *God Spoke to Me*

I lost just over 45 kilos. It took me about a year all up and I
hit about three plateaus along the way. At the Healthy Body
Club, plateaus, just like the ones I experienced, are the points
at which people begin to think they are never going to make
it to their weight loss goals. You feel as though you are
working hard at eating healthily and exercising, but the
weight will just not move.

Now I'm going to come clean here: plateaus are hard things
to come to terms with, and they can be hard to budge, too,
sometimes. But you can get through them, and the only way
to do this is by sticking at it. *Do not give up*. The only option
is to keep going. Surviving and moving beyond the dreaded
weight loss plateau is the difference between sitting on top of
the mountain with your weight loss goals achieved, staying at
the same place, halfway up the incline and feeling frustrated
that you can see the pinnacle but can't (or won't) reach it, or
having to take the lift for the rest of your life by slipping back
to your old weight. Where do you want to be? If you'll excuse
the extended use of this metaphor, the view looks just fine
from on top of the mountain.

I remember feeling incredibly frustrated during my

plateaus, but Crusher kept reminding me that even if my weight wasn't going down on the scales, the hard work I was doing was still making a difference to my long-term health and fitness. Every bit of exercise I did got me a little closer to my goal. Every healthy meal I ate put me closer to my goal. Every time I treated myself with love and respect it put me closer to my goal. That is, my goal of being a normal, healthy, fit individual no matter what weight I was. So, I kept eating healthily, exercising properly and being nice to myself, and felt proactive and in control even though I felt I wasn't *ever* going to budge off a certain weight. But you know what? I did. Every time. And you will too, if you just keep at it. There are a few other things you'll need to do as well, but the crucial thing to remember is not to give up.

Everyone experiences a damn plateau at some point in their weight loss adventure. For some people it's within the first two months, often coinciding with the six-week freak out (often it's the cause of the six-week freak out). For others it may be at around the three month mark of steady, continuous weight loss. For people like me, it is the last five or ten kilos that seem absolutely impossible to lose.

What is a plateau?

I have a few theories on the dreaded plateau. As far as I can see, there are three ways of looking at it: one, your body starts responding differently to what, how much and when you eat; two, your body starts responding differently to the kind of exercise you are doing; and three, your brain sets up a kind of psychological barrier between you and your goals. For me, the last thing was the most important, but I had to understand and act on the first two before I could even attempt to crack it.

The bottom line, though, is that the plateau is a necessary evil. When you hit one, look at it as a kind of rest time for your body and brain. When we were young kids, didn't we all love to curl up with our blankies and teddies and have that wonderful afternoon nap after which we woke up smarter, taller and stronger? Well, that's what I tell my five-year-old who refuses to have a midday nap, anyway! In all seriousness, the plateau effect is quite literally a breathing space for our body and brain to 'regroup' before it can keep marching on with the changes we are making to it. For example, even though I lost weight slowly and consistently over a long period of time (that is, safely), at one point my liver was in distress because I had lost such a lot of weight, and my body simply refused to lose any more until my liver was able to cope with the change.

The dreaded plateau and food

When most people start in the Alfalfa Zone, they often cut down their calorie intake quite drastically. Similarly, when some people have been inside The Alfalfa Zone for a while, they continue to keep cutting back their calorie intake in an attempt to speed their weight loss up. Either way, the body can startle and presume it is going into starvation mode. It doesn't know the difference between weight loss and famine.

I know I've banged on about this before in the chapter on fine-tuning, but I really need to ram this point home: if you decrease your calorie intake too much your metabolism *will* slow down: you won't burn fat, your body will eat your own lean muscle instead, and you will then start to stockpile fat. (Let me point out here that your heart is also a muscle, so don't do it to yourself.) Your weight loss goes nowhere – you hit a plateau. This is because your body needs regular, consistent amounts of healthy fuel and it's unsure of when it will get enough again.

I know from painful experience that it's extremely attractive, after changing your eating habits and losing a bit of weight, to start cutting back on meals and snacks in the hope of getting to your goal faster. If you get the urge to do this, remember that your new eating habits are a plan for life – there are no quick fixes that work in the long term and trying to get there faster will only put you back in your fat pants, eventually. In the meantime, you'll hover on the dreaded plateau until you decide whether to keep going in the healthy way, or keep going in the unhealthy way.

That said, once you make sure you are eating enough, you have to make sure that you aren't eating too much. Losing weight successfully, which means being able to crack the dreaded plateau, is a fine line between what you do and don't eat. A lot of people have great success in the first month or two; even though they have some major busts and revisit some of their favourite foods, they still manage to lose quite a bit of weight. But this is the honeymoon period. It doesn't last forever. The reason why you can lose so much weight while still 'breaking out' is because you have made so many changes to your input and output that your metabolism fires up and just burns, baby, burns. But once that settles down, it gets used to the reduced calorie intake and every little extra thing you eat starts ending up on your hips again. *Voilà* – the dreaded plateau.

When you hit a plateau, you need to ensure that you are eating often enough for your body to recognise that it's getting enough fuel, and also to start looking at your calorie and fat intakes in detail. You're going to need to fine-tune every meal, every snack, every drink and every situation where food is put in front of you. Usually, a short bout of focused eating like this will be enough to set your body off on the next lardslide. It won't be forever, but it does need to be for long enough to get you through the plateau. Going back to your food diary will help you do this. Now, some people, like me, may even have to cut right back on all treats, alcohol and fat just to get through the plateau. But remember, if this turns out to be you, it's not forever. You will be able to eat and drink those things again, but not while you're on the dreaded plateau (that is, if you want to get off the plateau and continue to keep losing weight).

Another plateau factor may be food boredom. You may be bored with always being 'good' or eating the same 'good' food – if this is the case, you'll need to start negotiating your treats or rewards with more zeal, and start introducing more interesting, but very low fat, food. Suffice to say that when you hit a plateau, using food as a reward or treat isn't going to help you. Start replacing the foods you are having as treats with non-food treats, like buying tickets to a movie or buying yourself a trashy magazine. Again, it's not forever, it's just while you're on the plateau.

I hit a plateau recently, and it lasted for three months. It nearly decimated my mental health, but I just refused to let it beat me. For some the damn plateau can be moved off in weeks, and for some it may take a month (or more) for your body to come to terms with its new, supercharged metabolism. But the main thing is that it will, and when it does, the weight will start coming off again. This is why you need to stay with it, and don't ever give up.

The dreaded plateau and exercise

Again, when you start in The Alfalfa Zone, the exercise you do really helps to keep that weight coming off consistently every week. But as you continue to lose weight, your body needs more and more resistance and challenge – the exercise you did when you weighed 100 kilos is just not going to work as effectively when you are 75 kilos. This is because when you were bigger, carrying that extra weight on your body was a workout in itself, but once it's gone you have to work harder and faster in order to keep the weight coming off in the manner to which you've become accustomed.

Chances are that if you walked your first 30 kilos off, you're going to have to run the last 20 off. I lost more than twice the weight of my child by walking and swimming. Just carrying Kai from the car into the house had my heart rate up – it still does. Imagine carrying that amount of weight on your body while you exercise (well, you can, if you strap a toddler to each thigh when you're on the treadmill).

So, when you hit a plateau it is time to really get moving. It is now time to exercise like you have never exercised before. Even though it sounds painful it's also hugely rewarding as you increase your level of fitness and start to achieve things you never thought physically possible. It's time to become the new you!

The other thing you need to recognise is that muscle weighs four times heavier than the same mass of fat (that is, it's denser), so while you may be losing fat and building muscle, it can look like a weight gain, or a maintaining of your current weight, on the scales. This is why it's so important to measure yourself – you may not be losing grams but you may be losing centimetres.

Also, if you're doing the same kind of exercise, week in, week out, your body gets used to it and stops burning fat as efficiently. Vary your routine, and surprise your body into fat burning mode again; and change the time at which you exercise. If you always get on the treadmill and then the bike, switch your routine around so that you do the bike first, then the treadmill. If you always go for a power-walk at lunchtime, start doing a jog at night. Keep your body guessing. And keep yourself guessing, or interested, too – it's harder to maintain a certain exercise if it is boring you. Try something new to keep yourself motivated. Do a class you have never done before. You might like it. You'll certainly like the weight loss when you finally crack that dreaded plateau.

The dreaded plateau and your emotional life

As you approach your goal weight you actually may be afraid of reaching it. What happens then, when you hit that magic weight? You may be afraid of losing control and putting all the weight back on; you may be afraid that you still won't be happy, or may still be single, or won't feel as successful as you thought you might be. Perhaps your weight has been the excuse you have used to be unhappy, or has been a distraction from the real issues you may be avoiding.

If this sounds like you, when you hit a dreaded plateau you may be sabotaging your own weight-loss success in order to avoid facing these issues. I know I did. Every time I reached the magic 10 kilo marker of 100, 90, 80, 70 and then 60 (I call it the naughties), I found myself self-sabotaging by bingeing, drinking more than I should or simply making bad food choices, thus preventing myself momentarily from hitting the 99, 89, 79 and 69 kilo markers of 'success'. I was particularly afraid of the power I would have when I got that sexy body.

One of the reasons why I stacked on the weight was for protection – when I was thinner I always felt as though there was a lot of sexual pressure on me. To be constantly sought after was difficult for me, and when you have trouble making people listen when you say 'no', or if you have been a victim of abuse, then it is a very scary thing to have to live in a body that a lot of people want a part of. But it's way more scary being lost in a body you can't control, and life is so much better knowing that you are not continuing that cycle of abuse.

If you think you are self-sabotaging your own weight loss, remember that you deserve to be healthy and happy and you *can* learn to deal with the new changes in your life. I learned techniques that kept the wrong kind of people away from me, without having to be fat. If you do the work on yourself, those psychological barriers will fall away and you'll realise that nothing is holding you back from reaching your goal.

Finally, I have to make mention of another quite common plateau effect which really hurts your weight loss. This is where you kind of diet but it doesn't work, so you give up and binge until the next week, when you kind of diet again, and then don't lose weight. You put on a kilo and decide diets don't work again, binge for another few days, promise yourself you'll never do it again, then starve yourself for three days . . . that is until you binge for another four days and then declare that you are a complete failure. This is otherwise known as the 'Am I ever going to start' plateau.

The reality is that diets *don't* work and there is nothing to 'start' but the rest of your life. And no, you are not going to get it right straight away. It's like expecting a baby to walk without ever falling down. You will fall down – often – and it will hurt, but if you keep getting straight back up again, you will get better at it. Recognise that you'll never be perfect because *no-one* is perfect.

You have to ask yourself if you are indeed ready to lose the weight, because unless you're ready to deal with the emotional aspects of changing the way you live your life, you will always revert to the days of old where pizza is your best friend, and everyone of the opposite sex can go to hell . . . because if they loved you they'd love you fat or thin. The real crux of the matter, though, is whether you love *yourself* fat or thin. If you are killing yourself by overeating then there's not a lot of lovin' goin' on, is there? I hate to use a cliché, but if you don't love yourself, no-one else can. I know it's true because I have lived that nightmare. It's not about what size you are, it's about how you treat your body and how you feel about yourself. If you get that sorted out you are going to be just fine . . . and you will crack that plateau!

With all these things in mind, here is my list of things to try when you hit the dreaded plateau.

The pep talk

Keep going. Crusher said to me 'Think of your fat as a velvet curtain. All the work is going on behind that curtain and when it is time, the curtain will fall away and reveal all the hard work you have done.' Remember that hard work is hard work. It does pay off. You may not be losing weight but you may well be losing centimetres. At the very least you are improving your cardiovascular system and therefore increasing your chances of a long and healthy life. (Unless, of course, you are destined to be killed in a plane crash, in which case it's better to have a good looking corpse that will fit in a normal sized casket, rather than your family having to buy two ground plots and a coffin that was once the cardboard box for a freezer.)

Control the food

- Keep your food diary. Make sure you are not suffering from food amnesia. If you're still telling yourself that food you can't remember eating has no calories, you won't crack the plateau. Analyse every day, week or month, and see if you can identify any patterns of overeating, bad choices or not eating enough. If you can see a problem area, focus on it and fix it. Add up your fat and calorie intake each day for a week. You might be surprised about what your intake is.

- Ensure you are eating regularly: breakfast, snack, lunch, snack, dinner, snack. Your body needs to know it's being fed, so that it can give itself permission to burn fat.

- Make sure you are eating enough. *Do not* skip meals. Don't cut back on the correct portion sizes of your breakfast, lunch, dinner or your snacks. Make sure you are getting the right serves of healthy food each day. Cutting back on food will slow your metabolism down and only make your body store what you do eat as fat.

- Make sure you are not eating too much. Make the best food choices possible. Watch out for extra helpings or extra snacks. Cut out all the butter and margarine, alcohol, mayonnaise, sugar and full-cream milk in your coffee and tea. Cut out cheese as well if you think it'll help you crack the plateau (but only give dairy up to get you through this difficult period – you need calcium to prevent osteoporosis). All these littlies add up and get stored as fat. Fatty foods in particular are converted into fat much more easily than protein. The body has to change the composition of protein before it can be stored as fat, thus burning up calories on the way. But fat is very similar to body fat and is stored with very little work.

- Eat breakfast within half an hour of waking. If possible, start getting up earlier and eating breakfast earlier. If you wake up at 7 am but potter around or nap till 9 am, change your habit. Get up when you wake up, and eat breakfast. You can go back to bed, but eat first. Eating fires up your metabolism which will help burn your way off that plateau.

- Cut out high sugar and high GI carbohydrate snacks, like muesli bars and low fat sweet muffins, and eat fruit instead.
- Similarly, avoid sports drinks, soft-drinks and fruit juices and other sugary drinks (including 'diet' drinks, because they get you used to the sweet taste), and drink water instead.
- Watch your carbohydrate intake, particularly at night (I don't wholly subscribe to this theory but in general it is worth a look at when you are trying to crack the plateau). Substitute high GI foods with low GI foods.
- If you don't eat enough during the day you are more likely to overeat at night – the worst possible time to do this. If you must eat sugary or fatty foods (it's not going to help your plateau, though) eat them earlier in the day when you have a chance to burn them off. And if you do eat sugary or fatty foods, *make sure* you burn them off.
- Drink lots of water. At least one litre, two if you can. It's easy to slack off on this. Your body needs water to function efficiently. In particular it stops your body from retaining fluid (which is no good on the scales and the plateau) due to dehydration. Drink!

Control the exercise

- Increase the intensity of your work out. Increase your heart rate to 80% of your maximum. Where you would normally walk for forty minutes, break it up by walking for three minutes, running for two and then walking for three again. Slowly build it up until you are running more than you are walking. Apply this increase in intensity to any kind of exercise you are doing, no matter what it is.

- If you work out at the gym, turn it into a circuit class. Do ten-minute workouts on the stepper, then ten each on the elliptical runner, rower, treadmill and the bike. The idea is to work harder for ten minutes than you would by just walking for forty minutes.

- Add an extra session of cardio to your weekly workouts.

- Change your exercise routine. Don't do the same thing at the same time; mix it up. Surprise your body into burning fat in a new way. It challenges your body and also relieves any boredom you may have from doing the same thing.

- Challenge yourself and step outside your comfort zone. Do a dance class, do a new gym class or join a sports team. There's nothing like the spirit of competition to get your arse moving!

- Set up an obstacle course in your backyard: sprint up and down, and do weights, sit-ups, push ups and skipping at either end.

- Walk as often as you can – to work, to the pool, to the video shop, to the supermarket. Walk your kids everywhere. Get off the train, bus or tram one stop earlier and walk the rest of the way.

- Walk and run with a friend and race them to certain points: to the nearest tree, to the bridge, or to the spunk 100 metres ahead. Short bursts of speed are better than no bursts of speed.

- Hire a personal trainer. They make you work harder than you would normally. Tell them to really kick your bum into action, and ask for a fat-burning program you can do in between sessions or at home.

- Lift weights; they will tone your ever-changing body, help avoid loose skin and the best thing of all is that muscle burns fat by just being in your body.

Control the mind

- Get some therapy. If you're frightened of reaching your goal weight, if food is controlling you, if you feel out of control, if you don't have the self-esteem to manage healthy food choices or to manage how you feel when you reach your goal, seek counselling. No amount of weight loss will fix deeper underlying emotional issues. And on a dreaded plateau, you will only hold yourself back. Get some help.
- Measure yourself once a month. You may not weigh less, but there may be a change in your shape. Let this motivate you to keep going.
- Read inspiring books about successful people you admire to keep you focused on your goal.
- Listen to motivational CDs and/or tapes every day. Learn self-hypnosis techniques (*Change Your Life In Seven Days* by Paul McKenna is great).
- Redo your anchors. Change them to focus you on your new short-term goal of getting off the dreaded plateau.
- Whenever you feel like crumbling, or are about to be exposed to temptations, repeat your next 5 kilo-goal weight to yourself: 'I am 79, I am 79'. This can really focus you.
- Set yourself short-term, fun fitness goals: half-marathons, fun runs, group walks. They'll keep you going when you feel nothing else is happening.
- If you can, stop weighing yourself, or throw away your scales. If you're using them too much, they mess with

your head. Remember, a muscly, fit 70 kilos is far better than a soft, squishy and floppy 60 kilos.

- Keep in mind that the plateau does not last forever if you just keep at it. Put one foot in front of the other (but just do it a little more quickly!).
- Remind yourself how far you have come. Pull out your fat photo and tell yourself that you have come a long way. Also, reward yourself for an honest week's work – treat yourself well during this time (but not with food).
- Don't give up. Even if you falter, don't ever give up!

Stay motivated

- Read your pledge every day. Put a smaller version in your wallet. Put it in the photo section so that every time you open it you see: *I commit to being the very best that I can be. I deserve to love, be loved and most importantly of all, I deserve to love myself. I deserve a healthy body and I will never give up on myself, no matter what happens, and I promise to do whatever it takes to make it happen. Today is the first day of the rest of my life. Shazam!*
- Write up your exercise routine in your diary. Check your diary every day
- Set your mobile phone alarm to go off when you promised you would go to the gym. Go to the gym
- Have a fat photo or a skinny photo on the fridge. Maybe even both
- Make a deal with a friend. Ring each other to motivate and support each other. Take turns each day. Make a bet and race them to your goal weight (with the maximum of 1 kilo loss a week). The winner takes all
- Each fortnight on a Sunday night, drag out your skinny clothes and try them on

- Before a night out, drag out your skinny clothes and think about how good you will look when you can fit into them
- Go shopping and try on clothes the next size down
- Constantly take time out to visualise your new, healthy body.
- Break up your goals monthly, weekly and daily. Reward yourself often with non-food treats
- On your desk or fridge have a list of new, fun things to learn and do, like rock climbing, belly dancing, pole dancing, tap dancing, salsa, bushwalking, surfing, roller-blading, horse riding, ice skating
- Read slimming magazines, sports magazines, and health magazines. And don't forget the internet!
- Find one new low fat recipe each week – cook it and eat it
- See food differently – instead of looking at chocolate cake as something yummy you are not allowed to have, think of it as a plate of fat and unhappiness that you would rather avoid. See food as fuel only
- Remind yourself every morning that it's a whole new day. Put the past behind you. The quicker you move on, the closer you will get to your goals.

Quick Quiz

1. At the beach, when someone suggests a game of volleyball:
   a) You head in the opposite direction and rent your shadow out to busloads of sun-shy Japanese tourists.
   b) You think they have suggested a game of beached volleyball and waddle off in a huff.
   c) You put your bikini top back on, readjust your g-string and take up your position at the net.

2. When trying something new:
   a) It has to be deep fried.
   b) Well, aah, you just *don't* . . .
   c) You can't wait to start. You love the challenge, and, given that you are naturally athletic and talented, you are good – no, *great* – at everything.

3. Complete this line – 'Feel the fear and . . .':
   a) Run in the opposite direction.
   b) Eat until you feel nothing.
   c) Just do it anyway.

Mostly a: It might be time you stepped outside your front door. No, you can't drive to the mail box. And stop paying the neighbour's kids to walk the dog.

Mostly b: It might be time to try something new – like walking, or at least putting down the remote control. It's a new thing, you might like it!

Mostly c: Wake up! You're dreaming. By the way, you really shouldn't eat in bed – those Cherry Ripes can be a choking hazard if you try to eat them lying down.

10

Step Outside Your Comfort Zone

Challenge yourself

'Don't ask what the *world* needs – ask what makes *you* come alive
and then go and do that. Because what the world needs is people
who have come alive.'

Howard Martin

The best three things I have ever done are join a soccer team,
compete in The City to Surf 14 kilometre fun run, and start
dancing again. When I threw myself into all of these things I
felt afraid, uncoordinated, fat, unfit and not sure I would be
able to do any of it. But conquering them all had me feeling
fit, fantastic, fabulously athletic and unafraid to step outside
my comfort zone – well before I had reached my goal weight.

The City to Surf

The City to Surf was always something I was going to do
when I got fit or thin – whatever came first. It was like there
was another AJ – a fitter AJ – and I had to wait to become her
to do all the things I imagined she would do. I was approach-
ing it from the wrong angle. What I needed to be doing was
all those things that would make me become that other, different person. It's the same as saying 'I won't go to the gym

until I lose some weight first'. But the truth is, you need to look at it differently: if you get your fat bum to the gym you will lose weight sooner.

The funny thing about me finally deciding to do The City to Surf is that my comedy partner and I were always hired to entertain the participants at the start line. We would do our Beryl and Cheryl characters – two fat, tragic ex-Olympians. Lou would wear a fat suit, and I would wear myself. I used to say, 'One day, Lou, I am going to get fit and do this race.'

So when the race came around and I still wasn't the completely fit AJ who did these kinds of things, I thought about waiting yet another year until I would magically be able to do it. When I discussed it with Crusher she told me straight away that I'd be closer to my goal if I got off my fat bum and moved instead of waiting for the perfect time or the perfect body – both of which might never come. The worst-case scenario, said Crusher, was that I would actually get fitter and lose some more weight. OK, there was also the possibility of having a heart attack and dying, but Crusher's motivation made me determined to give it a go regardless of what the outcome might be.

I talked a friend into doing it with me, and when she started procrastinating about sending in her form, I filled it out and paid for her myself and sent it off just in time.

Knowing that I was about to do something as challenging as attempting to run 14 kilometres, I found I was much more focused in the gym the few weeks before the race. I would run for longer, and push myself that little bit harder. I was determined to improve my fitness and not be the last one over the finish line.

It wasn't until the week before the race that I completely freaked out. Who was I kidding? Fat chicks like me didn't do The City to Surf. Everyone who knew I was doing it (including me) wondered whether I would survive Heartbreak Hill, whether I would get a cramp or a dizzy spell, faint, vomit or have a coronary. I was so worried I decided to drive to the Hill and try it on for size a few days before. I did it in no time at all. It was tough on the legs and it had me breathing a little more heavily but it was just not as bad as it had been made out to be. (Of course, I hadn't done the eight kilometre lead up to it, but I planned to overcome that obstacle on the day.)

The race itself was an experience I will never forget and one I feel compelled to return to each year now. First of all there is nothing like 'racing' down the streets of Sydney with 70,000 other people. It was such a visual feast: there were people in gorilla suits, fairy costumes (mostly men), families dressed up as 101 Dalmatians, numerous wigs, and lots of face paint and party frocks. It wasn't until the starter gun went off that I remembered to be nervous.

I set off with a run. The plan was to run as far as I could, then to run and walk as far as I could, and then finally to walk what was left. The first kilometre was downhill so that was easy. There was a bit of a steady incline after that, but it was downhill again shortly after that. I managed to keep my pace for the first four kilometres.

The five to eight kilometre section was a bit of a blur. I ran until I was puffed and then I would walk. When I recovered, I ran some more but I was slowing. My feet were hot and my legs were chafed (they were still fat enough to rub together). No-one told me that would happen. I started to wonder whether I would actually make it up the Hill. I was tired with seven kilometres still to go – and most of it uphill. I stopped to have a drink and decided to walk up Heartbreak Hill. Better to get there alive than to push myself beyond reason, I thought.

But halfway up that hill I found my breath and decided to

try running again. Before I knew it I was through the hardest part and pushing beyond the ten kilometre mark. There was only four more to go. I had blisters on my heels, my feet felt white-hot, I was limping, my formerly broken ankle was severely swollen and aching, and my toes were so painful they were starting to go numb. But I simply turned my attention to the finish line. I told myself there were only four kilometres to go. I walked four kilometres on the treadmill at the gym most days. I was going to do it. It was a matter of pride.

The crowd had thinned out by now and I was starting to pass people who had started in the pack earlier than me. I was overtaking people. I decided to run a little bit more. I did the Cliff Young shuffle – small awkward steps, arms locked in by my side and a slow but steady movement forward.

With only three kilometres to go my chafed legs were stinging and bringing tears to my eyes. I had to drop back to a walking pace, and my gait had me looking like I'd been horse riding (or got extremely lucky the night before!). I just wanted to finish. I was well and truly over it by then, and a part of me wished I hadn't done it at all. I stopped to put Band Aids on my now bleeding blisters, thought about Band Aiding my thighs and decided to just get there as quickly as I could. I decided to run again.

The rest was all downhill. That, in itself, was too good to be true. I had two kilometres to go when I heard this strange noise. It was a constant crunching sound – a bit like marching. I didn't know what it was but it matched the pace of my now heavily beating heart. I ignored it and threw myself towards the end, limping badly but telling myself the end was near. I came down the hill to discover a sea of plastic cups on the ground. The crowd was running over them, making the cacophonous crunching sound I had heard.

One kilometre left: I was on the final stretch. The end still seemed so far away. I could see it, and a guy collapsed in front of me, but I knew I wasn't finished yet. I stopped to help but was told by the ambos that he'd be fine in their care and to continue on my way. I wasn't sure I could, though. Completion wasn't guaranteed, even if I could see the finish line. I felt like telling them to follow me just in case I didn't make it but decided to save my energy for the very last stretch.

Despite feeling like my legs could fall off, I decided to *run* the last kilometre no matter what. I wanted to be running when I went over the finish line and I realised I wasn't the only one. Most of the people around me broke into a run and I put my pain aside and kept pace with the people around me. I was running – I couldn't stop. People were cheering, I looked out for Kai but couldn't see him (his godmother and he didn't make it in time – they expected me to cross the line later than I did. So did I).

I pretended everyone was cheering me. I pretended I was one of the first few over the line. I pretended I was not in the most pain I had ever known before – outside of the broken leg, of course. I pretended I still had some energy left and I crossed that line, filled with the pride of a girl who had decided – and subsequently proved – she was fit and healthy enough to do this race. A girl who was no longer, and would never be again, obese.

That first race was my coming of age. I had faced my fear and I had succeeded. I had hoped to do the race in 140 minutes – I clocked in at 121 minutes. It was no record breaking time but a personal best for me. It was my first ever race and I came 30,431st. I beat over 30,000 people. My legs felt like jelly and I knew if I stopped moving I might never get up again, but I felt the biggest high I'd ever had. I was filled with endorphins and immediately vowed to do the race the next year in less than 100 minutes (I did it in

99 minutes). Recently I completed the Sussan Women's Fun Run and ran the entire 10 kilometres in just under 70 minutes – only two years after my first City to Surf.

Two days after that first race I learned what happens when you don't stretch before or afterwards – your legs seize up. I was going up and down stairs sidewards, or on my bum (which was also sore) and went through so many ice packs there was an Eskimo knocking at my door asking me to go easy on the stuff. But I know I walked taller for weeks after the race and now it's an event I never miss – I'm always trying to improve on my time. And to help me through it all is that Nike slogan: 'If I can do this, I can do better.' That is how I have learned to live my life.

Survival guide for fun runs

Shoes: If you are going to run, you need good quality, comfortable, well-supported running shoes. You'll need to invest some money otherwise your feet and your back will pay. I recommend going to Athlete's Foot and getting a footprint done. They'll tell you what kind of shoe you need to buy with the right kind of support for your needs. Think about getting added support with gel soles, or extra cushioning. Every little bit helps. Then you can shop around and get the best price. You need to buy new shoes at least six weeks before a race or walk and you need to break them in (for tips on breaking in new shoes, see page 78). Do not wear new shoes on the day!

Wear good, soft, 100 per cent cotton socks that are fairly new. Perhaps even wear two pairs of socks. The last thing you need are socks that keep slipping down into your shoes.

Training: Start training as soon as you can; also, it's never too late to start. You may not have exercised for years but don't be put off. If I can do it, anyone can. Make sure you have a check-up with your doctor first; let them know what you are intending to do.

Start walking. Fun runs are not so much about fitness or winning – they're about endurance. Your legs are what will suffer the most so you have to build up their strength. Do lots of squats and calf exercises.

If the race is proving to be a psychological barrier for you, do a practice run a few weeks before the big day. As often as you can, visualise yourself doing it and walking or running confidently over the finish line. Do this every night before you go to sleep, especially the night before.

Injuries: If you have any previous injuries (like a broken ankle or leg) make sure you support them. Go to a physiotherapist the day before the race and get them to strap your old injury professionally. It will only cost you around thirty dollars and it can make all the difference between finishing the race or ending up at St Vincent's with a sprained ankle. Wear ankle and knee support bandages if you need them, and if you suffer from blisters stick Band Aids everywhere you are likely to rub. Put Vaseline on any areas that may chafe (thighs, knees, groin). Prevention is better than cure.

The night before: Get a good night's sleep (if you are too excited have some chamomile, or a Sleepy Time tea), eat a healthy meal (pasta is good), and don't drink any alcohol (it will dehydrate you and increase your levels of fatigue). Set your alarm clock to give you enough time to move at a leisurely, relaxed pace. You don't want to be rushing to the race. Take your time.

What to drink and eat on the day: Don't change your eating habits on the day of the race. Make sure you eat well by having a good breakfast and lunch, depending on when the race is. A banana smoothie and toast or cereal are a good start to the day. I always take a banana and eat it as I wait for the start of the race to give me an extra energy boost. If you are diabetic make sure you've had your insulin and sultanas to help you along. Avoid tea and coffee as they dehydrate you. Drink plenty of fluids a few days before as well as on the day, however, don't do what I did – I drank three litres before the race and spent half my time lining up for the Port-A-Loo. Drink three or four glasses of water prior to the race, and top up your fluids throughout.

Warm up: Stretch and warm up while you are waiting for the race to start. This will avoid pulling any muscles on the way.

The race: Listen to, and respect, your body. Top up your fluids throughout the race at every drinks station. If you get dizzy, see spots or start having an asthma attack, stop and consult with the St Johns ambos. Rest, recover and then go on unless you've been otherwise advised. If for some reason you can't go on, there is always next year. You have achieved a great deal by stepping outside your comfort zone and entering the race. Just do your best. That's as much as you can do.

Find someone with an equal level of fitness and agree to stay together no matter what happens. This buddy system really helps because the second-last kilometre is a killer, and it's good to have someone with you. You could even try training with them, to encourage each other to stay focused on your goal.

Have a support group at the end of the race. Running over that line is the mark of great personal achievement. Push yourself to do something you have never done before. For me, The City to Surf was my 'coming out' party. It was the new me. I reached the promised land well before I ever expected to, and suddenly the world was full of other fantastic opportunities. As I've said, the second-last kilometre is a killer, but the last one is a little easier because the finish line is the sweetest thing you have seen all day. Having friends and family there to cheer you on and take photos will give you that extra little push to really go for it. Even the people who walk all the way usually end up running over the finish line.

Take a disposable camera and have your race buddy run ahead and take a photo of you crossing the line. Then they can go back and do theirs while you record their moment of glory.

Fun run checklist

- Do lots of training before the event. Go for lots of walks – at least one or two the same distance you have to cover on the day
- Get your gear out the night before. Make sure you have everything you need. Nerves can make you forget important things, like a bottle of water, so do it when you are fresh and focused
- Eat breakfast and keep your fluids up before and during the race
- Take a jumper for the early morning cold and for after the race
- Apply sunscreen and wear a hat
- Pre-arrange to meet your loved ones. Don't rely on mobile phones. If there are a lot of people doing the race, the usage is so high mobile phone carriers get blocked or overloaded, signals go down and you can't get any coverage
- Push yourself
- Have fun!

Have your escape plan already organised. Think about having a friend drive in two hours after the event (you'll be starving afterwards so you'll want to eat first!) and pick you up and take you home. Or hire a limo to take you and your friends home. If you make it fun, it won't feel like exercise.

After the event: Keep moving, stretch and warm down, and keep drinking fluids. Also, eat well. Don't use it as an excuse to eat up, or eat junk. Reward yourself with a lovely meal out, or pack a sandwich to have at the end. Perhaps organise for your support people to bring a picnic.

Have a nice, long hot bath that night and don't forget the Dencorub. Think about getting a sports massage the day after. You will be sore for days, so remember to stretch and take it easy on yourself.

Soccer

That Nike slogan 'If I can do this, I can do better' applies to soccer for me as well. Team sports had always been a personal nightmare when I was growing up. Recently I wrote a children's book called *Blubberguts* (Hodder Hotshots) and it's about the fat kid who never gets picked to play on the team. That was me. Team sports meant ritual humiliation and bench sitting. When I discovered the school newspaper was put together in the sports periods an illustrious career in writing was born.

However, when my friend Tara lost all of her pregnancy weight in one season of soccer I thought it might have some extra health benefits for me, too. Surely that was worth a little ritual humiliation? What I didn't know then was that soccer would turn out to be one of the greatest joys of my life.

Every year I learn something new and get a little bit better. I started off as a goalie and have since scored many game-saving goals as striker (the position David Beckham plays).

The best part about it is that it doesn't feel like exercise. It's just too much fun. During winter I am the only one of my friends who not only doesn't put on weight but also takes it off. And that feeling of total body exhaustion has become one I look forward to because I know I have done an honest day's workout. You can't cheat on a soccer field because you have ten other people depending on you to do your best.

When the ball comes my way there is usually a girl half my age running for it. I may not get to it first but I always give it my best shot. I have all my team mates cheering me on. There is no way I would run that fast on the treadmill – no way in a million years – but I will do it every Sunday for an hour and a half, especially if there is a goal I can score, or stop being scored. Not only do I play willingly, I love every single minute of it, and my eating is so much more focused in the days following a game.

Soccer is the fastest growing female sport in Australia, which makes it really easy if you've never played before. Just join a team with women who are also beginners and learn as you go. If you're over thirty-five then join a team for over thirty-fives. They do exist and it is never too late to change the way you live your life.

I was on a team that didn't score a single goal for the entire season. But boy, did we have fun. And yes, the shorts were scary at first, but you soon discover there are women of all different shapes, sizes, ages, skills and fitness levels. The real key is to have fun – something I can guarantee *will* happen.

I can't wait till Sundays come around. The game really is the highlight of my week. Best of all Kai comes and plays with all the other kids (we call our team The Breeders because we're all mums, some with three or more children). He stands on the sideline, genuinely excited by the game, and proudly yells out 'Go, Mummy!' It's great for him to see me having fun and keeping fit. Sport is such a big part of our lives these days that I know he will never have a problem with his weight like I did. We all go out to the pub afterwards (near where we play there's one with a kids room and playground!) and have a relaxing post-game get together. I feel more alive than I have ever felt before playing soccer.

Dancing

I had grown up doing ballet, jazz and tap dancing. I never had the stick insect body to become a dancer but I loved it anyway. Even as an adult I continued classes, but when I became anorexic I stopped because I barely had the energy to get out of bed. Then, when I moved into the land of bulimia and obesity, I dropped out of acting as well. By then I was well into my cycle of self abuse. I think about it all now and often wonder whether I would have spent the next ten years being miserable, unfit and unhealthy if I had somehow kept dancing and got some psychological help way back then.

Like doing The City to Surf, going back to dance classes at the Sydney Dance Company was the one thing I was going to do when I got to my 'perfect weight'. At around the mid-seventies kilo mark I realised that there was no such thing as the perfect weight (or life) and I could either continue to half-live my life by feeling like a 'failure' about the things I didn't think I was able to do, or I could step outside my comfort zone and start embracing the things I love and had always dreamed of doing.

So off I toddled to Sydney Dance Company, the ultimate dance studio. I was terrified! It had been at least ten years since I had done so much as a pirouette, and the last time I did the splits was a year before on the dance floor at 3 am in a bad dance-off (which, incidentally, I didn't win. What I did get though was a double disc bulge, six months of not being able to exercise and an extra seven kilos back on my body. Sigh.).

With my heart beating wildly, I looked at my cottage cheese thighs and hoped the other dancers wouldn't try to dip crackers into me in the hope of getting a feed. But then I realised that dancers don't eat, so I swallowed my pride, donned my tracky daks and joggers and walked into the Beginners Jazz class. Despite having been a good dancer earlier in my life and having always taken the advanced classes, I realised that in the meantime there had been a dance revolution, I had aged, I was no longer as flexible or limber as I used to be, and my memory was not what it used to be. I was glad I was starting back at the beginning.

The room must have had at least eighty people in it. I hid up the back and was surprised to see women almost twice my age and even some people the size I was when I started my weight loss (110 kilos) so long ago. I silently high-fived those women and marvelled at their bravery. I wished I'd been able to do that.

The class started and the warm-ups were simple. Anyone could do it, and they did. I looked around with a bit more scrutiny. There were people of all capabilities and the egotistic dancer of my past held her head a little higher. I wasn't that bad after all. I sneakily pushed my way through to the middle of the class. Yes, there were plenty of those horrible dancer girls with great bodies (with no fat and great boobs – not that I was looking . . . OK, OK, I was), pony tails, pink clothes, pink shoes, pink socks and attitudes bigger than Melanie Griffiths' lips. Funny, that actually describes me when I was about seventeen. What a shame I always thought I was fat. Oh well.

The class moved on and we learned the routine. This is where it all started to unravel and I cursed all those joints I had smoked in drama college. Where was I? What was my name? What was I doing? What short term memory problem? That's right, I was trying to learn the routine. I have to admit my first class was extremely messy. And I guess I should mention that the teacher was one of the teachers I had had ten years ago when I was skinny. He hadn't aged a bit. It was like some weird scene from *Death Becomes Her*. Had he sold his soul to the devil when I had sold mine to Colonel Sanders? Double sigh. I hoped and prayed he wouldn't recognise me.

Just then, everyone did a double pirouette and I did what could only be described as an upright belly flop closely followed by an epileptic body roll (and I am allowed to say that because I have epilepsy. Don't write me letters!). My teacher did a double take. 'AJ?' he asked. I wanted to run and hide. I wanted to say 'No, my name's Sarah Jane Smith. I've never heard of an AJ' or 'Yes, it's me, but I've had a baby and that's why my arse is so big. I've suffered to repopulate Australia'. But instead I tripped trying to do the next step, lost my place and had to stop to get my breath back.

It didn't matter in the end. He didn't care. I'd been fat in dancers' terms back then (which wasn't actually 'fat' anyway) and I was still a bit chubby now. Whatever, I reminded myself. At least I was doing something about it; at least I was doing something I love. At least I was actually living my life rather than waiting for my weight to be perfect before I actually did the things I wanted to. In the end I had a ball.

I laughed a lot, mostly because I couldn't get the steps right, and even when I did everyone was already three steps ahead of me. It didn't matter. It was a hoot.

Every time I went back I got a little bit better. I'm no Mikhail Baryshnikov (thank God for that) and I'm still not up at the front of the class with all the snooty girls, I'm still somewhere near the middle. I still don't always get the steps right and I still don't have the perfect body. I may never have that, but at least I'm happy, getting fit and having fun. These days I do tap as well, and best of all Broadway Jazz, where the frustrated musical theatre performer in me gets her moment to shine. Watch out, Renee – *Chicago 2* is mine!

I always walk taller coming out of those dance classes, and almost skip to my car feeling a good deal happier and maybe even a little bit thinner. Best of all I know I am living my life to the fullest. It was something I waited far too long to do. You can step outside your comfort zone, too. You'll be amazed at what you can do and who you can be. Dare to be all that you have ever wanted to be. Dare to do it now!

Go on, do it

A little while ago I put my back out on the dance floor and put on 7 kilos because I wasn't able to exercise for six months. I was also seeing someone at the time and the relationship eating helped add to this as well. I went through the whole 'I'm a failure, everyone will be looking at me, I'm too fat to go back to the gym' thing again. It was especially hard because I was being touted as the world's newest 'dieting' queen. The reality is I am just a normal woman who lost a lot of weight and who has all the self-conscious body issues that every other woman has (and then some). It may take me a few more years to work out how to maintain my weight but when I do I promise to tell you everything!

Despite this, I woke up on my last birthday feeling depressed that I was back over 70 kilos after all the hard work I had done. I reminded myself that I couldn't help having injured my back, but that I could help the relationship eating, and the only way I was going to get back to my desired shape was to get my big arse down to the gym. I reasoned it was better to feel depressed about my body and be doing something to change it rather than feel depressed about my body and be doing bugger all about it. So, I set my alarm for 7.30 am on my 35th birthday and at 8 am I was running on the treadmill preparing myself for a hard class of Pump. Afterwards I felt fitter, thinner and feeling more in control of my life and my body.

Recognise that you don't have to wait until you get fit enough to do the things you've always dreamed of. If you start now, the fitness will come, and then it will come much faster after that.

Fun runs, team sports and taking dance classes are a great way to really push yourself out of your comfort zone, make you walk that little bit further, run that little bit faster and work that little bit harder. I took some of my weight loss club members in the Nike Women's Classic last year and one declared at the 8 kilometre mark that it was the best thing she had ever done. I knew what she meant.

There are plenty of charity walks and fun runs throughout the year, not to mention hundreds of team sport options (community, city, state and national events), and literally thousands of classes in all kinds of physical activity (dancing, martial arts, rock climbing, athletics – you name it, it's out there. Hell, you can even do pole dancing if you want!). Take the challenge yourself to do something new.

Just because you have never done it before doesn't mean you can't learn it. Simply set a date and book yourself in. You will absolutely love the things you achieve. The idea is not to think about it too much and get on with it.

Go on, do it, I know you can.

Challenge yourself

- Make a decision to change your life for the better
- Make a list of the new things you want to try, and try them
- Find a friend to do these new things with
- Sign up to a team sport and make new friends
- Focus on the fun, rather than the fitness. The fitness will come if you have fun
- Listen to your body
- Get the right equipment
- Try the hardest you can. Then try some more.

Quick Quiz

1. Your kids:
   a) Are so overweight they only ever get picked to be the mascot for the school soccer team.
   b) Eat take-away once a month and would like to have it more often but you won't let them.
   c) Only ever eat alfalfa, bean sprouts, mung beans and tofu, and are getting used to their New Age names of Apple Seed, Dill Pickle and Peanut Shell.

2. Your house:
   a) Is so full of junk food Greenpeace picket it as a toxic waste site.
   b) Has a little junk but is mostly filled with fresh fruit and good food.
   c) Is a junk food-free zone, as is your family's entire diet.

3. Your neighbours:
   a) Have renamed your place The House of Lard and charge people to look through the windows for $5 a pop.
   b) Often send their kids over to get a healthy home-cooked meal.
   c) Haven't spoken to you since you tried to sue them for polluting your air with barbequed meat smells wafting over the fence.

Mostly a: All-you-can-eat restaurants lock their doors and pretend they're closed when they see you and your family coming. Better fill out a donor card – for everyone. But don't bother getting any health insurance . . . none of you will be around long enough to use it.

Mostly b: Liar. You wouldn't be reading this book if you lived like this. Refer to a, above.

Mostly c: You need to eat some meat, stop channelling your psychic giant's inner child and start living in the real world. Ever heard of prohibition? It doesn't work. The first thing your kids will do when they move out of home is buy a fast food joint and eat their way to a heart attack.

11

Fit Kids, Not Fat Kids

Obesity and what it means for your children

'Seek not to make them like you.'
Kahlil Gibran, The Prophet

Why kill your kids?

I knew I was a big girl. I always (publicly at least) tried to make the most of my fat. I created some delightful fat comedy characters, like overweight ex-Olympians from the Beached Volleyball event; I wrote and sang powerful jazz songs about being big and beautiful; and I always showed off my breasts to their best with figure-hugging corsets and sexy low cut tops. But I was so busy calling myself a goddess that I didn't realise what was really going on. Deep down inside I knew that one day I would try to get healthy; I just wasn't sure when. I think I was waiting for that elusive, magical Oprah Winfrey willpower to kick in. I'd checked on eBay but it wasn't for sale yet, so I simply kept eating and drinking and telling people that I didn't care that I got stuck in the children's slide at Hungry Jack's.

I eventually realised that I'd been conning myself, big time, when I did the 'fat is fantastic' publicity stunt at Sydney Town Hall – the defining moment was when the only media crew who turned up wanted to interview me, not because

I was the fat, funny chick who deserved her own comedy show, but because I was *obese* and happy to stay that way. Having that word applied to me had an immediate, horrifying impact. 'Obese' was not just fat, 'obese' was the word you heard when people use a crane to get lifted out of their house. Gilbert Grape's mum was obese. Marlon Brando was obese. People died of obesity. Being obese meant I was at risk of diabetes and all its associated life-sapping symptoms, as well as heart disease or, worse, heart failure.

I suddenly realised I could actually die from living the way I was. And considering I was a single mother of a small boy with *no* family support, the fact that I was his only life-line hit a painful nerve. It was one thing to ruin my own life, but to defiantly risk ruining his was a different matter altogether. I looked at him and noticed he, too, had double and triple chins. I was making him fat. I remembered the horrendous teasing I got at school . . . and I wasn't even fat then! I knew how it had affected me and I knew I couldn't consciously continue to keep feeding him unhealthy food. The teasing would be the same for him, only worse if he was actually overweight.

Now, Kai and I live a healthy life together, and I know I have probably given us both ten to fifteen years of extra living and a better life in general because we aren't overweight any more, and we are really fit. (Kai often does his little hand weights when I do mine, and he's always trying to show people his 'huge muscles'.)

There is so much talk about adult obesity in Australia as our national rates skyrocket towards those of America. But sadly, the rate of obesity in our children is mounting – fast – and it's just as frightening. Almost 25 per cent of our children are obese and the figures are increasing, pardon the pun.

As parents, it is time to take responsibility. Do not under-estimate the impact that being overweight will have on your kids. Ask yourself: do you truly want to do that to them? I know it'd be a perfect world if everyone was treated equally, but put the indignant outrage aside and think of the health issues. When your kids leave home they can eat what they want, but while they are under your care it's your job to do the very best that you can to teach them about healthy living. It might take a little more work but it's far better than watching entrenched bad food habits destroy your child's life.

The problem is that it's just too easy to buy convenient, quick fix food, and/or to reward them with rubbish. There's also so much peer group pressure on your kids to eat the same foods as their friends, and clever child-focused adver-tising makes it almost impossible not to make that food seem attractive. There never, ever seems to be enough time to cook a perfectly well-balanced meal, so you find yourself reaching inside the freezer for yet another heat-'n'-eat dinner of fatty, non-nutritious crud. But the truth is that unless you accept that fresh food is best and that you do *not* want to make your children fat, you should never rely on this stuff to feed the family.

Don't kid yourself that they'll grow out of the fat, either. Children with one or more overweight parents are much more likely to be overweight themselves; and overweight children are enormously likely to become overweight adults. The research and statistics consistently show this to be true. And we know now that being overweight puts you at risk of developing type 2 diabetes, heart disease, as well as all the associated complications of these diseases. As well, a child who has been obese is more likely to develop cancer later in life. Also, let's not forget the awful, long-reaching emotional repercussions of being an overweight child. There is the low self esteem, the teasing, the non-inclusion in activities, and the inability to participate in sport with ease. Why give your children a sense of failure before they even establish a sense of their own self? Why kill them slowly when there is no way that you'd choose to kill them quickly?

Think of it this way: if I handed you a needle and said, 'Inject your child with these diseases that will significantly reduce the length and quality of their life', would you do it? Of course the answer is a resounding 'No!' Then why do it at all? No matter how long it takes, the diseases associated with obesity will kill you. Don't pretend that chubby kids are just little jolly balls of joy. Being overweight can seriously affect their health and their length of their life. On top of the brainwashing that comes with some fast foods (here's a toy for eating this meal, doesn't that make you feel good?), don't add your own brand of influence to it before they have a chance to learn to live and eat well themselves. Why make it harder for your children to make healthy choices because you are unhealthy, or worse, healthy but still feeding them crap?

Manage your children's food

Don't get me wrong, though. I'm not saying that we should never eat take away food and that your kids should never be allowed to have their lolly bags. It's a fact of life: children will eat this kind of food whether you're around or not. In our family Kai has his fair share of junk, but we have rules and he is aware of the consequences of what he eats – good or bad.

Kai was actually four before he knew what McDonald's or Burger King was. He came home from his Noona's house with a toy, telling me about this great place called McDonald's. The next week he stayed with someone else and hit Burger King, and, as he called it for the next few weeks, King Burger was firmly planted in his head as the greatest place on earth with its very own playground. How could a healthy ham, cheese and tomato sandwich compete?

I've only just relented on the cordial front. Kai is five now and we've only just started having it in the house. He drinks watered-down juice in the morning and water or milk the rest of the time. On weekends he can have cordial but not in the morning or at night, which really only ever gives him a couple of hours of opportunity. He's never had Coke and only ever has lemonade on very rare occasions. The good thing is that he doesn't really like it because he's not used to the bubbles. He says it's 'too spicy'.

When Kai gets a lolly bag (I usually halve it in size; and no, I don't eat them . . . well, maybe just a few . . .), he's not allowed to eat it all at once. He is allowed to keep it in his room, though, because he knows and accepts the rules about when to eat junk, as we call it. He knows he is not allowed to have lollies or chocolate in the morning, except of course on Easter morning and only even then after breakfast. We also have drive-through rules: he can only have it once a fortnight at the absolute maximum, and he has to have done some sport or physical activity beforehand.

Kai has a firm understanding that junk food is something he can't have all the time; and that if he did, he'd be unhealthy. On the odd occasion that he does pester me for a packet of chips as a snack, he has to eat 'real food' first, like an apple, banana or a sandwich. The wholesome food is good for him, as well as fills him up, and generally makes it impossible for him to eat a full packet of chips. It also gives me an opportunity to educate him because when I say he has to eat 'real food' first he always follows it with a plaintive 'But why, Mummy?'

I then explain that apples are good for him and have vitamins and minerals that help him grow stronger and smarter, and that junk food is just that – completely meaningless as a food; that it doesn't do anything good for him. Sure, I could deny him the chips, but again, prohibition doesn't work and all I'd be doing is making that kind of food more elusive and attractive because he's not allowed to have it. All he'd do when he leaves home is become the CEO of Fatty Snackfoods Australia, just to spite me.

I'm really mindful of never using the words 'special occasion' or 'treat' as this conjures up the idea that those foods or drinks have some kind of positive connotation and are then sought after. I do say 'Just this once', though. When Kai asks why he can't have the food all the time I tell him that it's bad for him in large amounts. When he asks why other kids have it all the time I tell him that their mummies and daddies aren't looking after them properly (well, all right . . . I actually say their mummies and daddies don't love them enough. Yeah, I know it's harsh, but it's not the worst thing I will do as a mother!).

The great thing is that, occasionally, when people offer Kai an unhealthy food he comes out with, 'But that's junk food. My mum says that junk food makes you fat if you have too much.' Every now and then Kai will actually pass on the junk food or lollies declaring, 'I only want to eat healthy food now, Mummy. I don't want my teeth to fall out from too much sugar and I want to live for a really looooooong time.' That usually results in a few extra stars on his chart for being such a grown-up boy. Of course, that doesn't mean he doesn't also chuck a major wobbly when I have said he can't go to Maccas. We have those days as well!

Every now and then when we are out and Kai throws a tanty, some lovely old lady or shopkeeper offers him a lolly 'to make him feel better'. I always politely decline, which usually forces the tanty up to warp speed, but I reckon accepting the lolly is dangerous training, emotionally. In that scenario the lolly means happiness or comfort. I suffered from this and ended up with an arse bigger than England, then had to spend ages with a shrink working out why I reach for food when I'm feeling down. Lollies and chocolate only ever make us feel better if we have been taught that. Why give your children food addictions that might take them half their life to get over?

You'll probably find those same positive reinforcements of unhealthy food all through your childhood, too: 'If you clean your room you can have an ice cream', 'If you be a good girl I'll give you a lollipop'. They sound benign enough, but they're not. If you are going to give your kids an ice cream or lollipop, just give it to them and don't overload them with positive reinforcement. Don't attach a feeling of achievement to the food. When you reward your kids for doing great things, give them pocket money or stick a star on their star chart. I use both of these systems in our house. Kai can save up his pocket money to buy a new sword or a magazine; and when he gets enough stars on his star chart he can have what we call a Kai-day, which means he can choose what we do that day (like go to the zoo, go cycling in the park etc). He's learning the value of money because he has to save up for things he likes and wants, and isn't getting an ingrained sense that bad food is a reward for him being good.

Eating healthy food should never be painful or feel like a punishment. I had a severe hatred of all vegetables, and still do despite actually liking the taste of some of them. The emotional baggage I carry with me about the humble veggie has been one of my greatest obstacles to getting healthy. I spent many, many nights of my childhood sitting at the dinner table until late at night; I wasn't allowed to leave until I ate my over-boiled vegetables. On a few occasions I was actually made to eat them . . . so there are no surprises as to why I developed a major phobia. Don't make your kids suffer like that. If they don't like the taste of something, find a way to cook it so that they do. Kai 'hates' mushroom and zucchini, both of which are hidden away in his spaghetti bolognaise, which he would eat seven times a week if he could. I also make up veggie soup and stick in some two-minute noodles and he is more than happy to eat that, too. Dr Jenny O'Dea, a Sydney University nutritionist who has carried out extensive research in child nutrition, suggests that sometimes children have to try something up to ten times before they like the taste, or are just used to the idea of it. Don't give up – keep offering them good, healthy food. Eventually it will stick: they will like it, and you will have succeeded in teaching them about healthy food choices.

I know it feels like a battle most nights, but it's just not worth getting angry with them if they don't want to eat everything on their plate. In her book, *Positive Food for Kids*, Dr O'Dea also recommends that you, as the parent, should decide *what* they eat, and the child should be allowed to decide *how much*. Her research shows that children know how much they need to eat in order to satisfy their hunger. So, if you force them to clean up their plates when they have already satisfied their hunger, you are only succeeding in teaching them to overeat. If you want to teach them about the starving kids in Africa, send the money you're saving on the food bills off to sponsor a child instead. It's a much better life lesson.

Also, be aware that you may be imprinting your own, idiosyncratic cravings on your child. I have to work against doing this all the time. To this day I wrestle with the habit of buying the petrol and chocolate to go with it. Even when I'm aware of it I find myself buying the treat for Kai instead of myself. That way I'm not buying it for me and it won't hurt if I just have a little bit. I also do it with hot chips; I ask Kai if he wants some (and of course I can always depend on him to say yes), so that I can steal one or two, but generally three or four and/or most of them. But we need to think of it this way: if we're not buying them for ourselves because we know the food is unhealthy, we shouldn't be buying them for our kids either. Don't teach them that it's OK for them to have the food, when it's not healthy enough for you. If you do it all the time your kids end up with mixed messages about eating healthily. Leading by example is extremely powerful. As the parent, *you* are the person your kids look to for guidance on how to live their life.

Kai asks me why I don't eat ice cream or have dessert or eat chocolate very often. I tell him 'Because I don't want to undo all the good work I have done.' I'm always mindful that he looks to me as his role model. The other day someone asked Kai if he remembered what I used to look like. He replied, 'She had a big fat bottom, a really big belly, and bosoms that looked too big.' He then followed it up with, 'But now she's going to live till I'm old enough to marry her.' Sigh. My work is done.

But don't be misled; I'm certainly not perfect, and I'm not a food Nazi, either, so he has a little of everything but he knows there are rules and consequences of all he eats and does.

With all this in mind, here are some tips for encouraging healthy eating for your child:

1. Label foods as 'sometimes' food and 'real' food. It helps to create a firm image of what is good and not so good for them.
2. Also, try not to call lollies and chips a 'treat'. Use the word 'junk' – because that's what it is. It helps prevent positive reinforcement of unhealthy food and teaches your children to have a dietary conscience.
3. Employ the 'real food first' rule: for example, if they are going to have a lolly or chips, they have to eat something good first, like fruit, a sandwich or yoghurt.
4. For snacks, package up baked pretzels, dried fruit, apricot bars and sultanas in lolly bags. It looks fun and makes your kids feel special. You can try putting a small, cheap toy in there as well so they look forward to morning tea.
5. Don't use butter or margarine on your kids' sandwiches. They just don't need it; neither do they care; in fact they probably won't even notice you've stopped using it. The earlier you start this the less likely you will have to retrain them in later years. When you're using jam or peanut butter, don't use butter as well. If they resist total change, just butter one side of bread. After a few hours of it being in their lunch-box they won't know whether you've buttered both sides or not. Then try and cut it out altogether a bit later by using a little bit less each week.
6. Offer your kids the drive-through cash-back deal: if they don't pester you for drive-through food for a month they can spend the saved money on whatever they want at the toyshop or bookshop.
7. Water down their fruit juice. It has lots of natural sugar (fructose) which translates as extra calories they don't need, and also which can cause problems for their teeth if they're not cleaning their teeth often enough or well

enough. Water it down when they're not looking and do it slowly – don't do half and half in the first week; do a 1:3 ratio at first and see how you go.

8. Instigate a rule about drinking cordial and soft drinks on the weekend only.

9. Don't punish your children because they have trouble eating vegetables. Be patient, be positive, keep telling them about the amazing health benefits of the food, and keep serving it up. As Dr O'Dea recommends, sometimes kids need to have food put in front of them ten times before they'll eat it.

10. Make a star chart with a line for each new fruit and/or vegetable. Every time they try something they get a star, as well as high praise. When they fill the line with ten stars allow them a present like a small toy. (Do not offer them a food reward.) 'It's a new thing. You might like it,' became a big catch-cry in our house.

11. When they move beyond the tasting/accepting star chart, make up another star chart for their recommended daily serves of fruit and vegetables. If they fulfil their weekly quota, reward them with things like inviting a friend over, or going to a movie . . . whatever fits in with your lifestyle. Just make sure the rewards are things you can sustain!

12. Never create incentives with junk food. If they clean their room when you ask them to, give them a star on their 'help around the house' chart, or 'good behaviour' chart. When they get a certain amount of stars, again, reward them for good behaviour with whatever you think fits the bill, as long as it's not food.

13. Keep healthy snacks in the glove-box of your car for when you are out and about without any food and they are 'starving'.

14. If your child refuses to eat 'real' food, don't give them sometimes/junk food (usually this is done to make yourself feel better that they have eaten at least something). If they are really hungry they will eat what they are offered. If they don't, they're driven by something else other than hunger, like a craving, boredom, a need for comfort or habit. Remember the recognise-challenge-distract method for figuring out why you want to eat from earlier on in this book? Use it on your kids, too.

15. Don't fill your kids up with food or drink before meal times, particularly dinner. If you can, try and leave at least an hour of no eating before each meal. If they are really hungry, give them a piece of fruit or some yoghurt. Make eating good food a priority.

16. Never say never. Prohibition only makes the banned food seem more attractive. A little of everything is the way to live a healthy, balanced life.

17. Find healthy alternatives to favourite sometimes/junk food. You can buy low fat hot dogs, low fat ice cream, low fat lollies, low fat chips, and low fat fat. Well, maybe not the last one, but almost everything has a low fat option or alternative so there really is no excuse.

Manage your child's exercise

Exercise is essential for a healthy life but it also should be fun, particularly for kids. One of Kai's great joys is our end of the day walk. During the summer it is a nightly event. We eat our dinner and then go for a long stroll through the neighbourhood, trying out new streets, and tip-toeing past churches where dragons are sleeping in the cellar. In winter we meet friends on the weekend and take a walk around the harbour or local bay. We always stop at the playground at the end, provided Kai has walked and not relied on the stroller. We have a special deal: no walk – no playground.

I had a lot of mother guilt when I was getting fit. Kai would stand at the edge of the soccer field, crying and screaming for me. It was the same at the gym. He would always turn on a tanty whenever I put him in the crèche. Of course, as soon as I was out of sight he was fine, but he made sure I felt really bad before I walked out that door. He would always say, 'But why, Mummy, why?' I would hug him and tell him that I was getting fit so that I could live longer and spend more time with him. Now, Kai's used to the amount of exercise I do, and now runs ahead of me, joyful that in words that are now his own: 'I'm going to run, Mummy, so I can get fit and live longer'.

I eventually switched soccer teams (and clubs), travelling an extra half an hour, because I found a team filled with mums. We all bring our kids to the games and although it's a little bit like *Lord of the Flies*, the kids run around in a big gang and have the time of their lives. We go to a kid-friendly pub after the match and they are all now the best of friends. Exercise is now a part of our life together. Kai knows I am committed to staying fit and he has that desire too. He can't wait to go to his swimming classes, or Little Athletics, or martial arts every week, and is always running, running, running everywhere. He also understands that exercise is good for helping you lose weight if you need to: every time I get off the treadmill (which is in our lounge room) he sits on my lap, presses my tummy and declares, 'See, Mummy, you're not fat any more'. The other thing he does of late is check the state of my fadubadubas (chicken wings), declaring that they're actually shrinking. How cute is that? I love him so much I could eat him. Hmm . . . maybe not.

First lead by example, then get your kids into a sport they love. Get them to try as many things as they can until they find the one activity they absolutely love. Be supportive of their need to find something they can do well and enjoy; don't force them to do something they hate – it'll only ever make them hate exercise, or team sport, or guys with whistles . . . or the creepy mascot! Make sure they're not being picked on for being the last one around the oval, too. I quit playing hockey in high school because I was made to do 100 sit-ups and three laps of the oval for being the slowest one around. That was the last school sport I ever did, managing to land the job as the editor for my school newspaper. A writing career was born and my big arse began to grow.

The great thing is that most organised sports will either let you do a session free or have a reduced rate for trial sessions of around two to three weeks duration. You don't actually have to buy all the gear only to discover that the next week your little darling hates soccer and wants to do baseball with his best friend, but then somehow manages to find out about how great gymnastics is. Stay patient and encouraging and remember that it doesn't matter what the sport or physical activity is, as long as they do something.

I really also want to stress that it's important not to focus on your child winning or being the best at their chosen sport. Let me share a story with you. Kai has been doing Little Athletics for a little while now, and he pretty much always comes last or second last in every race he takes part in. I make a big point of telling him the hare and the tortoise story, and we always focus on him doing his best and trying his hardest, rather than focusing on where he comes in the race.

Recently he formed a really lovely friendship with the other little boy who also comes last or second last. This boy's dad always makes a big fuss about them crossing the finish line, rather than where they were placed, and tells them that anyone who finishes is a winner.

A couple of weeks ago, this boy's dad pulled off his son's shoes and showed Kai and me his feet. Jasper had thick scars running all the way around his ankles and toes. He'd had years of painful reconstructive surgery and rehabilitation on his feet, and was told he would never walk . . . yet here he was doing Little Athletics.

That day, he and Kai ran a long race. All the other boys streamed ahead. Kai was well behind the group, and so was Jasper, who was starting to limp. Eventually it looked as though Jasper wouldn't finish the race, but my beautiful little boy ran back to him, put his arm around his friend's shoulder and helped him along till they ran across the finish line together, three minutes after the winner, but with the crowd cheering them on. Then Kai declared they were winners that day simply because they had finished. There wasn't a dry eye on the entire oval! That week I bought the boys trophies for displaying the best team spirit. They were so chuffed!

Focus not on how many times your child wins or who they can beat, but on who they become as little people. Triumph of the spirit is the best gift you can give a child – it'll stand them in such good stead for the rest of their lives.

Children are sponges. They learn what we teach them, so teach them to honour their bodies. If you make health and fitness a way of life then they'll never have to undo damage or re-learn how and what to eat, or struggle with accepting that exercise is so important for their bodies. I wasted so many of my years hating myself for stuffing my face with

rubbish and doing no exercise and the physical consequences that went with that, when I could have been having
the time of my life on the soccer field or in The City to Surf.
Oh for the power of foresight!

Here are some tips for getting your child more active:

1. Get your child involved in a team sport outside of school
   activities, or enrol them in a gym fitness program aimed
   at children.
2. Walk them to and from school/preschool/day care.
3. Pay them to walk the dog; or organise them to walk the
   neighbour's.
4. Never yell at them about their game or sport (from the
   sidelines or not). Always be supportive and positive.
   Never be angry or punish them if they don't play well or
   make a mistake. Always praise them for their effort, no
   matter what it is, and remind them that tomorrow is
   another day.
5. Go for family walks as often as you can.
6. Use the television as a reward for good exercise. For
   example, if they play outside for an hour, they can watch
   their favourite show.
7. Let them see you being active and fit. Take them to see
   you playing your sport or doing your exercise. Explain
   the great benefits of being fit (you live longer, are
   happier, are more active, can play with them more).
8. Never force them to do something they don't want to.
   Understand and accept that some kids like to swim, and
   some like to run: everyone's different. Make an effort to
   help them find something they love to do.
9. Always reward your child when they do well at their
   sport (and also when they don't). Make them feel fantastic for doing their best – no matter what the result.

Reinforce that they are gaining so many health benefits from just taking part.

10. Teach them to understand that competition is good because it helps them strive to run faster or better, but that winning isn't everything. Being healthy and fit is.

Don't underestimate how important it is that you teach your children about good health and fitness. The unconquerable high self esteem they'll get from putting all they know into practice will get them much further in life than being able to recite their times tables accurately. I firmly believe that making your children fat or obese is child abuse. If you knew you could make your child obese in thirty seconds you wouldn't do it . . . So don't do it slowly.

Treat their little bodies with the love and respect they deserve. Let them fulfil their life's potential unburdened by an overweight body and a distorted view of what food really is. Teach them that food is fuel and the body is something they need to nurture and take care of to carry them on what will hopefully be a very long journey through a wonderfully fulfilling life.

Help your kids live healthy lives

- Start cooking the same healthy low fat meals for your kids
- Be honest with yourself: if you wouldn't eat the food you serve your kids, don't give it to them
- Set food boundaries and stick to them
- Limit their junk food by having rules about when they eat it, and don't keep it at home
- Find a sport your child likes and get them playing it
- Do lots of family physical activity, like going for walks
- Remind yourself that it's your job to give them the best opportunities for a healthy life
- Give them a healthy life – while you're at it, give yourself one, too!

12

Final Word

Make your dreams come true

'The difference between millionaires and billionaires is that millionaires read their goals once a day and billionaires read theirs twice.'

AJ's life coach

By the time you are reading this chapter, hopefully you have started your weight loss and fitness adventure, and have already lost a kilo or two. If this is correct, you're well on your way to becoming fit, healthy and as happy as Barbie in her dream house (tee hee!).

What do you mean, you're still eating chocolate? Put it down, and get moving. Don't be the one who gets left behind. Other women are taking control of their lives and heading for the gym right now. It really isn't as difficult as you think. Yes, it can be tough, but not as tough as living your life hating yourself. Just commit to changing your life for the better. Decide to do it, and then just do it. Henry Ford said, 'Whether you think you can or whether you think you can't, you are probably right.' Decide that you *can* become a healthy person, and start living like a healthy person. It doesn't matter that you don't believe that you are a healthy person for the first little while – soon you won't even be thinking about what you can and can't eat, and what you can and can't do at the gym – you'll be making healthy choices because it has become a habit, and maybe even because you enjoy it, too.

However, you won't be able to make change in your life until you are ready. No-one else can make you ready. You have to want this more than anything else in the world – yes, even more than chocolate. But when you *are* ready to do this, the most crucial thing to remember is *keep going*. No matter what obstacles appear, you *will* get there. Try not to look at bumps in the road as failures, look at them as learning experiences. And never let anyone get in the way of making your dreams come true. Listen only to your heart (and me). Keep reminding yourself what you are aiming for, and keep going – every time the sun comes up, treat it as a new start. Your dreams will become a reality sooner than you think.

Now let me tell you a story. I have always believed in being able to make my dreams come true by using creative visualisation. Basically it means that if you want something to happen, you must believe that it is *already* so, thus it *will* be so.

When I quit my extremely lucrative job in radio, I made a very hippyish pact with 'the universe': I would follow my dream and whatever I believed to be my destiny (it was to become a writer), and the universe would provide for me. I remember being absolutely terrified leaving my job and going on the dole (sorry, I mean the John Howard Arts Scholarship for Promising Writers) – I had always had enough money in my life till this point, and I had absolutely no idea how I was going to support myself and my young son. I decided that I hadn't been specific enough in my request to the universe, and decided that what I needed was a $15,000 grant from The Australia Council to write an album of spoken word (poetry). Flipping forward in my diary a few months, I wrote on the entry for 3 October: 'I receive cheque for $15,000!'

I filled in my application form and sent it off, fully believing that I'd win the grant. Every day, every week and every month that passed I looked at that diary entry and repeated it as a mantra. But two weeks before that portentous date, I received a letter from the Australia Council telling me my application hadn't been successful. I was shocked and devastated, felt betrayed and ripped off – and afraid. I had just been evicted, and had no money at all. My son and I were about to become homeless. I began to question my entire belief system – I just couldn't believe things hadn't happened the way I'd planned. They always had.

But then I gave myself a good slap. I told myself to get real. Everything else had always worked out for me, so there was no reason why it wouldn't work this time – I was just going in a direction I was un-used to, or hadn't thought of before. So, I laughed in the face of 'literary merit' and sent off the first two chapters of the book I'd been writing in my spare time, *Confessions of a Reformed Dieter*, to an agent. Within a week I had signed a book deal, and on 3 October I received a cheque for $15,000 from my publisher – the very same day I had written it in my diary. *Confessions* became a bestseller, and since then I have had a few more book deals; one, a kids book called *Blubberguts* (about a fat kid who comes good), and of course this guide to losing weight and getting fit. I reckon my whole literary career was allowed to blossom because of those five powerful words I wrote in my diary.

So (yes, I have been leading up to a point . . . and here it is), in order to become fit and healthy, you must *believe* that you are fit and healthy, and then you will become it. This is why I say 'bluff it until you become it' until I'm blue in the face. At some time in the future, in the midst of puffing and panting on that treadmill or climbing up those stairs, you will get a rush of endorphins or experience the high of being able to do it without feeling like you're having a heart attack, and then you will want to do more. And when you do more you will achieve even more highs and successes, which will fuel you further towards your goal. Suddenly, at some time in the future, you will be a fit, healthy person who has taken control of your compulsions and has transformed your life.

If you write your goal down and look at it often enough, it becomes a part of your everyday thinking. If you say it out loud often enough, you will start believing it. And if you believe it, there is no option: you will become it. It's the same as that 'build it and they will come' way of thinking. Oh dear, I'm sounding a bit New Agey. I'd better go have a joint, eat some lentils and sit in a Kombi for a while. (Damn, I don't do drugs or have a Kombi, not to mention lentils not being high on my to-eat list. Sigh.) But seriously, this is why it's important to have a body goal. It gives you a clear idea of what you want and keeps you focused on achieving it. You can do it for all aspects of your life but it's particularly successful for health and fitness issues.

Here is a visualisation exercise that may well help you on your way. It certainly helps me. First of all, have a brainstorming session and identify all the things you want to achieve. For example, it could be to find enough time to work out at the gym or go for a walk. It could be to run 7 kilometres in under forty minutes, or to do a fun run or marathon. It could also being able to fit into your skinny jeans, or being able to squeeze your bum back into the swings at your local park. Whatever they are, write those goals down.

Next, turn all of your goals into one single powerful and meaningful statement, a personally empowered pledge to yourself. Give it a time frame, too. Think big, but make sure it's achievable. It's pointless saying that you'll will go from a size 26 to a size 12 in six weeks. It just won't happen. Well, not without killing yourself in the process, anyway, or ending up a size 28 two months later.

Most importantly, your pledge should be written in the present tense. To help yourself do this, look to a time in the future when these things will be a reality. For example, *It is 1 January, 2006.*

Then say how you feel: *I feel fantastic. I feel so alive I am constantly surprised. I have so much energy, my skin is glowing, my hair is healthy and I skip through my days with boundless enthusiasm.*

Now be specific: *I weigh 65 kilos and am a healthy size 12. I have a toned, trim, healthy body with great muscle definition and very sexy calves. I not only fit into my skinny jeans but I bought my first mini skirt.*

Describe how you want your life to be: *I run 7 kilometres three times a week in just under forty minutes. My body does this with ease and I am invigorated and amazed that I am still cutting my time down. My soccer game is improving and I have been named player of the year. I do weights twice a week and have great muscle tone to show for it. I am strong, healthy and athletic. My health is at its peak.*

Make sure you cover everything: *My eating is in control and I simply love all the healthy food I can now cook without having to refer to recipes. I am more confident than I have ever been. I manage my time well and always make sure I have enough to exercise. Everything runs smoothly in my life because I am on top of things.*

And finish big: *I adore my sexy new wardrobe, love all the attention I am getting. I feel more alive than I thought it ever possible to be. I am on fire! Contentment, peace and happiness are mine.*

Be careful to keep your language positive. For example, instead of writing *I am no longer in pain. I am not over-worked. I am no longer stressed,* word it more positively: *My body is strong, healthy and I move with the freedom of an athletic person. I feel calm, confident and able to tackle anything that comes my way. I am strong, capable and happy.*

Early last year, after fighting my way back from an injury, I got back into the swing of things by doing a creative visualisation. Here it is:

It is 1 November 2004 and I feel fantastic. I am on top of the world. Today I weighed in at 60 kg. I am trim, taut, (fake) tanned and terrific. I have an abundance of energy and am the healthiest I have ever been. I run three times a week and have achieved my goal of doing 7 kilometres in less than 35 minutes. I have great endurance. I am strong, fit, well defined and have only 18 per cent body fat. My skin, hair and nails are vibrant, healthy and stronger than ever before. I eat healthy food every day and I am in control. I am focused, confident and brimming with self-esteem. I love my new leather boots that zip all the way up my sexy, defined calf muscles. My tight bum looks great in my skinny jeans. I love my new wardrobe filled with size 10-12 feminine, sexy dresses. Kai and I have the most loving, giving, caring relationship and we are ecstatically happy in our active, healthy life. I am inspired, happy, content and just love to be me. Shazam!

Once you have written your pledge, make it look as lovely as possible (print it out, decorate it), and put it somewhere you will read it at least twice a day (the toilet door is an excellent place). Read it as often as you can, and believe it is so. Those words will become a silent mantra and will help you powerfully on your way to becoming that healthy person.

Now that you have set your body goal and written your pledge, I do want to reinforce that getting to a size 10 will not fix all your problems. Fixing your problems, though, *will* help you get healthy and fit and to a size you are happy with. Don't be afraid to face your demons. Get professional help if you need it, or find reliable emotional support in the form of a friend or family member if you think you're not ready for that step. Whatever you do, never underestimate the weight of unresolved emotional issues. Getting healthy on the inside will help you get healthy on the outside. If you take that first brave step towards being the person you've always dreamed of being, chances are you're determined enough to get there.

Remember, you deserve a healthy body. You deserve to be fit and active. You deserve to love yourself and treat yourself well. You deserve to look in the mirror and like what you see. You deserve the very best friends who support you in whatever you do. You deserve to love and be loved. You deserve the very best that life has to give so go out and settle for *nothing less than the very best.*

Just take it one day at a time, an hour at a time, and if you need to, a minute at a time. But be gentle on yourself, and forgive yourself. Treat yourself the way you would treat your own child; treat yourself well. And most importantly of all love yourself.

I thought I was a lost cause. I had given up on myself and I never imagined I could change my life the way I have. I am such a different person now. Not so much because I am a different dress size but because of all the work I have done on my compulsions, the way I look at food, the way I think and the way I see, feel about and treat myself. I am not perfect – not even close – but I am perfect in my imperfections and I love myself more than I ever have. Every day of my life gets better because of it.

Life is better than I imagined it could be. I love to run and play sport, and being fit and strong is the closest you can get to feeling invincible. I love the fact that my beautiful son Kai now lives a healthier life and, God willing, we will both live a longer, healthier, happier life because of the changes I have made.

You can too. Believe me when I say this: You *can* change your life for the better. You *can* take control of your life. You *can* have the body you want. And you *can* have your cake and eat it, too. Just remember that what we vividly imagine, ardently desire and enthusiastically act upon, must inevitably come to pass.

And if all else fails, bluff it until you become it.

Now go and get that body you've always dreamed of having. I'll see you in The City to Surf and on the soccer fields. And don't forget to say hello!

Shazam!

Your Food Diary and a Four-week Eating Guide

Food diary

Photocopy the blank pages on pages 280–1, and fill it in daily as your own weight loss and exercise diary. As you'll see from the examples following it is a great way to keep track of what you are eating, how much exercise you're doing and how you are feeling. Sometimes it's a bit of a shock to add up your figures and find those few 'treats' have doubled your fat intake for the day. Keep reviewing how you are doing and what and where you can do better. If you stay honest (that is, write *everything* down), remain focused, and keep reminding yourself of your goals you *will* achieve the body you want.

Food diary samples

Monday 27th January, Week: 1	
B: 2 slices of toast with peanut butter, coffee	**Cals:** 1900
	Fat: 80 g
S: 2 Tim Tams, chocolate bar	**Ex:** 45 min walk
L: Ham and salad sandwich, Coke	**H₂O:** 4 glasses
	Comments: *Very menstrual*
S: 10 jelly snakes, packet of chips and a hot chocolate	*and craving comfort foods.*
	Be more prepared tomorrow;
	will get a protein bar,
D: Lean Cuisine, glass wine	*diet chocky mousse, and fruit.*
S: WW ice cream	*Tomorrow is a whole new day.*
	At least I walked! But too
	much fat and calories.

Tuesday 28th January, Week: 1	
B: Cereal with skim milk, half banana	**Cals:** 1250
	Fat: 45 grams
S: Apple and yoghurt	**Ex:** 45 minute walk, 25-minute
L: 98% fat free satay noodles, kiwi fruit	swim
	H$_2$O: 5 glasses, plus three
S: Crackers with tuna, diet chocky mousse	lime cordials, one Coke and
	an applejuice
D: Healthy homemade pizza	**Comments:** *So proud of*
S: Fruit salad and Colombo ice cream	*myself. The tuna really got*
	me through to dinner without
	the usual arvo cravings.
	Wanted a Mars Bar but had
	diet mousse instead. Tasted
	great. I will be in my skinny
	jeans in no time at all.

At the end of each week, analyse the changes you need to make for the next week. For example:

Sum-up of the Week
More H$_2$O.
Less cordial and other drinks.
More fruit.
Less chocolate.
More salad.
Make sure I eat enough for breakfast.

Weekly weigh-in and monthly measuring

As well as weighing yourself every week, measuring your shape and size is a great gauge of checking how you are doing in your new healthy lifestyle, especially when you have hit a plateau and you haven't registered any change on the scales. Don't weigh yourself any more than once a week – if you do it any more than that, you're more likely to be disappointed with the results because your gains (I mean losses!) will be so small, as opposed to being pleasantly surprised most of the time. Try and keep it as a weekly thing so it doesn't mess with your head. Also, only measure yourself once a month, for the same reason. Here's a handy chart you can photocopy and fill in each week after each monthly measuring up.

Date:	Week:
Bust – nipple line (cm):	
Under bust – bra line (cm):	
Waist – belly button (cm):	
Hips (cm):	
Upper thigh – the widest (cm):	
Lower thigh – above the knee (cm):	
Arm – between shoulder and elbow (cm):	
Neck (cm):	

Monday	Week:
B:	Cals:
S:	Fat:
L:	Ex:
S:	H_2O:
D:	Comments:
S:	

Tuesday	Week:
B:	Cals:
S:	Fat:
L:	Ex:
S:	H_2O:
D:	Comments:
S:	

Wednesday	Week:
B:	Cals:
S:	Fat:
L:	Ex:
S:	H_2O:
D:	Comments:
S:	

Thursday	Week:
B:	Cals:
S:	Fat:
L:	Ex:
S:	H_2O:
D:	Comments:
S:	

Friday	Week:
B:	Cals:
S:	Fat:
L:	Ex:
S:	H_2O:
D:	Comments:
S:	

Saturday	Week:
B:	Cals:
S:	Fat:
L:	Ex:
S:	H_2O:
D:	Comments:
S:	

Sunday	Week:
B:	Cals:
S:	Fat:
L:	Ex:
S:	H_2O:
D:	Comments:
S:	

Sum-up of the week

Four-week eating guide

This is a very basic getting-started eating plan, particularly if you know that food planning and controlling portion sizes is difficult for you. Use it as a rough plan, and then gradually start making the changes you need to live your life healthily and in control, on your own. **Please note:** it is not my intention that you follow this plan meal for meal. It's simply a collection of ideas to show you the kinds of things you can eat, and how much you can eat, and still lose weight.

I'm a creature of habit. For five out of seven days I have cereal and yoghurt for breakfast. The same goes for lunch: I have sandwiches or soup six days a week. I don't particularly mind any more that it's often the same kind of food. However, in the beginning it was really important to give myself some variety to keep it interesting, so this is where this plan is helpful.

I have included a lot of allowable 'comfort' foods in these beginning weeks, because if you are anything like I was I needed sweet treats and muesli bars to keep me going. These days I mostly have fruit or yoghurt as my snacks. The important thing is that you start with these 'better' choices and then move on to making the 'best' choices you possibly can.

So keep in mind that you don't need to have the snack (or dessert) at the end of the day – you *would* be better off without it. You also don't need the muesli bars – you *would* be better off eating fruit. You don't need the Lean Cuisines – you *should* have fresh food at all times. But this is the lazy girl's guide, so take it slowly and do the best that you can. If you want to replace all your snacks with fruit then go for it. If you want to learn to cook from week one, then do it. Remember, if you eat like a healthy person you will become a healthy person!

Week One, Monday

B: 2 crumpets with lite peanut butter, low fat yoghurt

S: Apple, banana

L: Lite ham and salad sandwich, 8 grapes

S: Peach, 3 red licorice strips

D: Lean Cuisine Chicken Satay Noodles and salad

S: Nestle Diet Chocolate Mousse, 3 strawberries

H$_2$0: 8 glasses

Tuesday

B: Cereal with skim milk and banana

S: Special K bar, apple

L: Chicken breast and salad on lavash bread

S: Fruit salad and low fat yoghurt

D: Grilled fish, spinach and ricotta pie and salad

S: Weight Watchers Mango Ripple ice cream, peaches

H$_2$0: 8 glasses

Wednesday

B: Low fat banana smoothie, ½ English muffin with diet jam

S: Sultanas and dried apricots

L: Sushi, apple and kiwi fruit

S: Low fat yoghurt, peach

D: Lean Cuisine and steamed veggies

S: Nestle Diet Creamed Rice, ½ sliced banana and 8 blueberries

H$_2$0: 8 glasses

Thursday

B: Cereal with skim milk, 1 sl toast with Marmite

S: Orange, 2 sl pineapple

L: Veggie soup and bread roll, frozen mango

S: Tuna on rice thins

D: Chicken stir-fry

S: Fruit salad and Weight Watchers ice cream

H$_2$0: 8 glasses

Friday

B: Low fat yoghurt, 2 crumpets with lite peanut butter

S: Two fruits pack, 1 small Caramello Koala

L: Bagel with smoked salmon, baby spinach, red onion, cream cheese, squeeze of lemon, apple

S: Handful of baked pretzels, 6 grapes and 3 strawberries

D: Homemade seafood pizza and salad, 2 glasses of wine

S: Nestle Diet Cheesecake dessert

H_2O: 8 glasses

Saturday

B: Egg white omelette with tomato, mushroom and lite ham, fruit frappe

S: Low fat strawberry smoothie

L: Toasted sandwich with tuna, Nestle Diet Chocolate Mousse

S: 1 sl low fat banana cake

D: Penne with tomato-based sauce, salad, 2 glasses of wine

S: Orange

H_2O: 8 glasses

Sunday

B: Poached egg on toast, grilled tomato, small gl orange juice

S: 2 Saladas with Vegemite, kiwi fruit

L: Pumpkin soup, 1 sl toast

S: 1 sl H_2O melon, 6 grapes, 10 blueberries

D: Homemade lean hamburger and salad

S: Weight Watchers ice cream

H_2O: 8 glasses

Notes

Week Two, Monday

B: Cereal with skim milk, mango

S: Rice crackers and low fat dip

L: Tuna, lettuce, onion sandwich, banana

S: Low fat yoghurt, apple

D: Spaghetti bolognaise and salad

S: 1 sl banana bread

H_2O: 8 glasses

Tuesday

B: Porridge with skim milk and blueberries

S: Low fat strawberry smoothie, 2 Weight Watchers cookies

L: Tuna and salad, half rockmelon

S: Low fat yoghurt, 4 jelly snakes

D: Honey mustard chicken, rice and steamed vegetables

S: Nestle Diet Chocolate Mousse

H_2O: 8 glasses

Wednesday

B: Boiled egg, 1 sl toast, 4 strawberries, small gl skim milk

S: English muffin with diet jam, low fat yoghurt

L: Chicken salad, banana

S: Apple, K-time Muffin Bar

D: Grilled barramundi and salad, glass of wine

S: Fruit salad

H_2O: 8 glasses

Thursday

B: Cereal with skim milk, low fat yoghurt

S: Special K bar, kiwi fruit

L: Lite ham and salad sandwich, fruit salad

S: Rice crackers and low fat dip, carrot and celery sticks

D: Lean Cuisine with steamed veggies

S: Low fat custard, banana and strawberries

H_2O: 8 glasses

Friday

B: 2 crumpets with diet jam, low fat yoghurt

S: Low fat strawberry smoothie, sugar-free Chupa Chup

L: Dolmio mushroom risotto, banana

S: Apple, kiwi fruit

D: 2 Chicken skewers, steamed veggies

S: Diet jelly

H_2O: 8 glasses

Saturday

B: Low fat bacon and egg roll, small gl apple juice

S: K-time bar, mango

L: Lite chicken caesar salad

S: Quarter rockmelon, 2 sl watermelon and 6 grapes

D: Roast lean lamb with oven-baked vegetables

S: Weight Watchers ice cream, poached pear

H_2O: 8 glasses

Sunday

B: Berry pancakes with maple syrup or lemon juice

S: Banana, low fat yoghurt

L: Focaccia with ½ chicken breast, lettuce, tomato, avocado

S: Sl low fat chocolate cake

D: Tom Yum seafood soup, 2 fresh pork rolls

S: Fruit salad, small gl skim milk

H_2O: 8 glasses

Notes

Week Three, Monday

B: Cereal with skim milk, banana

S: Kiwifruit, 1 Salada with lite peanut butter

L: Cup-a-soup, lite ham and salad sandwich

S: Apple, 3 strips red licorice

D: Grilled salmon steak, stir fried veggies

S: Nestle Diet Chocolate Mousse, 2 strawberries, 1 teaspoon blueberries

H_2O: 8 glasses

Tuesday

B: Muesli with low fat yoghurt and peaches

S: Banana, 1 low fat chocolate biscuit (Farmbake choc chip)

L: Miso soup, sushi box

S: 1 peach, 1 plum

D: Lean Cuisine and oven baked veggies

S: Gl wine, 10 grapes

H_2O: 8 glasses

Wednesday

B: Boiled egg on toast, ½ mango

S: Crispbread with prawn and avocado

L: Bagel with turkey, cranberry sauce and salad

S: Banana, low fat yoghurt

D: Oven-baked fish, spinach and ricotta cheese, and salad

S: Diet jelly

H_2O: 8 glasses

Thursday

B: Sultana bran with skim milk, 1 crumpet with lite peanut butter

S: Low fat muesli bar, orange

L: Pumpkin soup, bread roll, apple

S: 3 pikelets with smoked salmon, lime and dill sauce

D: Home-made lean hamburger and salad

S: Fruit salad

H_2O: 8 glasses

Friday

B: English muffin, low fat cream cheese, strawberries

S: Sultanas, 6 rice crackers, 1 sl low fat cheese

L: Chicken breast salad

S: Low fat yoghurt, peaches

D: Pasta with tomato-based sauce, 2 gl wine

S: Vitari ice cream

H_2O: 8 glasses

Saturday

B: Egg white omelette with ham, low fat cheese, mushroom and tomato

S: Low fat strawberry smoothie

L: Focaccia with lean turkey and salad

S: Pear, apple

D: Low fat home-made pizza

S: Low fat tiramisu

H_2O: 8 glasses

Sunday

B: English muffin, 2 rashers of low fat bacon, grilled tomato, small gl apple juice

S: Low fat chocolate biscuit, kiwi fruit

L: Veggie burger with salad

S: Wendy's Chocollo ice cream

D: Lean Cuisine and stir-fried veggies

S: Fruit salad

H_2O: 8 glasses

Notes

Week Four, Monday

B: Cereal with skim milk, banana

S: Fruit salad, low fat yoghurt

L: Pita pocket with low fat cream cheese, lite ham, lettuce, tomato, grated carrot, beetroot

S: Handful pistachios and almonds

D: Vegetable soup, 1 sl low fat home-made pizza

S: Low fat fudge brownie

H₂0: 8 glasses

Tuesday

B: 2 sl fruit toast, low fat cream cheese, banana

S: 15 low fat corn chips with tomato salsa

L: 15 cm baguette with low fat cream cheese, smoked salmon, red onion, baby spinach, capers

S: Peaches

D: Satay beef stir-fry

S: Orange

H₂0: 8 glasses

Wednesday

B: Berry pancakes with maple syrup

S: Apple, low fat yoghurt

L: Baked potato with lite ham, sun-dried tomatoes, lite cheese and mushrooms

S: Handful baked pretzels, sultanas

D: Veal steak with steamed veggies

S: Fruit salad with low fat ice cream

H₂0: 8 glasses

Thursday

B: Cereal with skim milk, mango

S: Low fat Moove chocolate milk, banana

L: Low fat pea and ham soup, bread roll, apple

S: 30g dried fruit 'n' nut mix

D: Spaghetti bolognaise

S: Nestle Diet Creamed Rice

H₂0: 8 glasses

Friday

B: Bagel with diet jam, low fat yoghurt

S: Apple, kiwi fruit

L: Chicken breast and salad sandwich

S: Orange, low fat muesli bar

D: Sesame beef skewers, ⅓ cup steamed rice, steamed veggies

S: 2 gl wine

H₂0: 8 glasses

Saturday

B: 1 scrambled egg, toast, orange

S: Apple

L: Chicken breast and salad

S: 2 sl pineapple, peaches

D: Grilled salmon steak with steamed veggies

S: Air-popped popcorn, 2 gl wine

H₂0: 8 glasses

Sunday

B: Fruit salad, low fat yoghurt

S: 2 Vita Weets with lite peanut butter, Cadbury Highlights Hot
Chocolate Drink

L: Low fat chicken noodle soup, lite ham and cheese sandwich

S: Pear, 1 sl low fat cheese

D: Roast veal, oven-baked veggies, low fat gravy

S: Banana, low fat custard

H₂0: 8 glasses

Notes

Twelve Weeks of Goals, Exercise and Motivation

'The only way out is through.'
AJ Rochester

Here's a twelve week exercise and motivation guide to help you through the first twelve weeks. Those early months are when you really need some extra planning and motivation. I had a lot of crucial weekly help from Crusher and Nutcase throughout my entire weight loss campaign, and I think it's important that you also find someone you can trust who will help inspire you to keep going, as well as working with this guide (if you want to).

When those first three months are up you'll be into the hang of things and will be freestyling your new healthy, fit life. The way to work with this plan is to read the goals, quotes and exercise parts at the beginning of the week, act on them during the week, and then read the motivation entry at the end of the week, when you really need a boost to start the next week. My advice is to photocopy the guide and wallpapper it where you won't miss it (the toilet door is a great place).

Week One

Goal: Your life changes the very moment you make a decision, so start now! In your food diary (see page 280) you have to write down everything you eat and drink, and how much exercise you do including walking and housework. Also write down how you felt and the things you struggled with. Do the very best you can do. Stick to regular meal times and if you do have a breakout, remind yourself of your personal pledge (see page xiv, or pages 273–74) and get back to making the very best choices that you can. Don't give up. Think about those skinny jeans you want to fit into next season, or next year. Don't think about the bigger picture; just take it a day at a time.

Quote: 'Procrastination means paying twice the price when you eventually must act.' (TA McAloon)

Exercise:
- Go for a brisk walk three times this week for a minimum of twenty-five minutes each time.
- Do the bum squeezes, tummy tucks, stair thingies and sit-ups every second day. If you want to do it every day, go for it. Just don't burn yourself out.
- Take the leap and join a gym. Think about doing one weights session (and do one if you can).

Motivation: Congratulations! You got through the first week. Yes, I know you thought about food every single minute of every single day, but that will change, I promise. And yes, I know it probably wasn't a perfect week but you have to focus on the changes you *have* made and congratulate yourself for being brave enough to start. Now, go through your food diary and circle all the times you had a breakout, and where you could have made a better choice. Try and analyse why these things happened, see if there are any solutions you can come up with, forgive yourself and move on. Promise yourself that, next week, you'll halve the amount of times you break away from your healthy eating.

And don't forget to do some exercise. Make the time, book it in and stick to it. No excuses.

Week Two

Goal: Do not skip breakfast. Get up ten minutes earlier if you have to, but you must eat within half an hour of waking. This week you have to start moving more. Drink more water and do not miss any meals. Stick to breakfast, snack, lunch, snack, dinner, snack. Remember the lolly rule (if you're going to eat it, eat fruit first). Try to limit your alcohol intake. Keep reading your goals, every day. Do the best you can.

Quote: Don't focus on what went wrong; concentrate instead on what you can get right.

Exercise:
- Go for a brisk walk three times for a minimum of thirty minutes each time.
- Do the bum squeezes, tummy tucks, stair thingies and sit-ups every second day. Do them every day if you can.
- Make sure you actually join the gym this week instead of thinking about it, and don't just dream about doing a weights session, do one.

Motivation: Good work. Make sure you do something nice for yourself for having got through the second week, like buying a lovely trashy magazine, or having a hot chocolate with marshmallows from the café (low fat, of course!). Set yourself a reward for when you hit the four-week mark (e.g. a facial, massage, pedicure). Write it in your diary and book it. Remind yourself you are creating *new* life habits, and habits take time to set in. Make sure you are eating enough at breakfast time, don't overeat at snack time, and don't have chocolate or lollies at night. Save them for earlier in the day so that you've got a chance to burn them off. Whatever you do, just keep going. You *will* get the body you want if you just stick at it.

Week Three

Goal: Make sure you're not missing your snacks – eat, and eat regularly. Keep your body burning, baby. Speaking of which, it's time to bump up the exercise. Stop making excuses, and follow the exercise plan below, or do one extra session of vigorous activity on top of what you're already doing. Focus on making your food choices better every day. Don't just have toast for breakfast – have cereal and yoghurt, or porridge and fruit. Make sure you eat *enough* fruit. But if you do make any bad choices, just start afresh at the very next meal. Don't wait for the next day to start. And keep going. You're doing really well.

Quote: As you risk failure you take two steps closer to great success.

Exercise:
- Go for a brisk walk two times this week for a minimum of thirty-five minutes. Do the bum squeezes, tummy tucks, stair thingies and sit-ups every day.
- Do one other session of cardio (a class at your gym or aqua) and do at least one weights session (do two if you can).

Motivation: What a great week. You're almost halfway towards making some permanent, life-long healthy habits (when you hit seven weeks you'll be *looking forward* to eating healthy food and will be *excited* about exercise). Picture your new healthy body and stay focused on that. Ask yourself what you want more: healthy habits and the sexy body, or the KFC and a bum the size of Canada?

Week Four

Goal: Cardio, cardio, cardio. Keep moving! You should also be getting really hungry these days, now your metabolism has woken up. Make sure you always eat enough to get you through to the next meal, and cut back on the alcohol. Try to have only two nights a week where you drink, and when you do, have only two drinks each time. It's also time to start refining or fine-tuning your eating a bit more. Substitute high carbohydrate snacks with fresh fruit and veggies. And join that gym if you haven't done it yet. The sooner you hit the gym, the sooner you will have the body you want.

Quote: The best way to predict your future is to create it.

Exercise:
- Go for a brisk walk three times this week for a minimum of forty minutes. Do the bum squeezes, tummy tucks, stair thingies and sit-ups every day.
- Do one more session of cardio (like a class at your gym or advanced aquarobics) and do at least two weights sessions (do them before your cardio class).

Motivation: Congratulations! Go and get your four week reward. You have now been in The Alfalfa Zone for a whole month, and you have your reduced size or weight to show for all your work. You're a legend. Yes, there are things you could have done better but look at all the amazing changes you *have* made. It's time to try on your skinny jeans. It won't be long before you're slipping them on with ease. Don't forget to do your measurements – they'll reflect all the hard work you have done.

Week Five

Goal: Don't slacken off. Just because you've lost some weight while still being able to have a few treats like chocky, lollies and chips doesn't mean it's going to continue. Your body *will* slow down its weight loss, so stay focused. Eat well and keep making better choices, and keep moving. Book in your 'good month deal' reward for the end of this month at eight weeks. What will it be? A weekend away, sky diving or horse riding?

Quote: 'If you dream it you can do it.' (Walt Disney)

Exercise:
- Go for a brisk walk four times for a minimum of forty minutes. Try the walk/run routine: run (i.e. jog) until you can do no more, then walk until you recover. Start over and keep doing it until the time has finished. Try and finish on a run, and then do a slow warm-down walk.
- Do the bum squeezes, tummy tucks, stair thingies and sit-ups every day.
- Do one other session of cardio (a class at your gym or

advanced aquarobics) and do at least two weights sessions (do them before your cardio class).

Motivation: Another excellent week. You're probably about to hit the six-week freak out in the next week or so, so be warned. It's absolutely normal, but make it easier on yourself by not beating yourself up if you have a big breakout. Just get it over with, and get back to making good choices. Perhaps give yourself some more food variety this week to stave off boredom and stick with your food diary so that you can see exactly what you're doing. Don't get slack and fill it in every couple of days. Fill it out during the day, or at the end of the day. You don't want calorie amnesia – snacking on things you can't remember. Always be honest with yourself. Are you eating as well as you can? Are you exercising as much as you can?

Week Six

Goal: OK, you're in dangerous territory. You're probably about to have a new, healthy life breakdown or freak-out. At the end of it all though, you'll be breaking up with Pizza Hut forever. It takes about six weeks to create new habits, so this week can be crucial in terms of setting your new habits in place for life. Try not to have a crash and burn; or, if you do have one, try to minimise it as much as possible. Nurture yourself. Keep your week simple. I know it seems as though it's been hard, but you *will* be allowed to have the things you enjoy, just not in the amounts you used to have. Exercise as much as you can this week because it'll keep your eating focused. Love yourself and remind yourself of your goals, every day. When you've got through this, your healthy habits will be set in concrete – perseverance will pay off!

Quote: 'Dream as if you'll live forever. Live as if you'll die today.' (James Dean)

Exercise:
- Hire a personal trainer to run you through a high-level cardio workout that you can do at home or in a park.
- Find a set of stairs (a big set) and run up them, and walk down them (safety first!) for thirty minutes.
- Go for a walk/run three times for a minimum of forty minutes.
- Do the bum squeezes, tummy tucks, stair thingies and sit-ups every day.
- Do one other session of cardio (a class at your gym or advanced aquarobics) and do two to three weights sessions (do them before your cardio).

Motivation: Hooray! You got through this week and you're still here; that's the most important thing. Yes, you could have done better and yes, you may still be daydreaming about food a lot, but at least you know now it's not the be all and end all. Look at your happy food list and make a healthy alternative of something you are craving. You are breaking old habits and creating far healthier ways of living your life.

Week Seven

Goal: It's time to get tough. *Stop* sneaking those extras. They are keeping you from reaching your goal. Start fine-tuning every aspect of your eating. It's time to give away making just better choices, and start making the best choices you possibly can. Make your house a safe place. You can't eat crap if you haven't got it. You'll be getting a bit bored around this time, so start learning some new recipes and make really interesting things to eat. Constantly challenge yourself. And wherever you go, never be caught out without healthy food. Be vigilant.

Quote: The world was not flat. It took Christopher Columbus to risk going over the edge to discover whole new continents. What is waiting around the corner for you? You won't know unless you make the move to go somewhere other than here.

Exercise:
- Go for a walk/run three times for a minimum of forty minutes.
- Do the forty-minute cardio workout the personal trainer gave you.
- Do the bum squeezes, tummy tucks, stair thingies and sit-ups every day.
- Do two other sessions of cardio (a class at your gym or advanced aquarobics) and do at least two to three weights sessions (do them before your cardio classes or at home with free weights).
- Do a video class at home (e.g. yoga or pilates).

Motivation: Ah yes, saboteurs. They tend to work a bit harder at around this time. Your body should be showing significant changes, but don't be surprised if nobody says anything, apart from 'Want some hot chips?' It doesn't mean they haven't noticed. Keep an eye out for the people who prefer you the size you were, and be strong. Don't let them influence you. You deserve a healthy body, and to be fit, strong and happy with who you are. Keep going. And if you do crumble, four steps forward and one step back is still three steps forward!

Week Eight

Goal: You need to start changing your exercise routine now by working harder and running faster. Constantly challenge yourself to work at a higher level. Yes, it is hard, but once you lose that weight you'll never, ever put it back on. It's worth some hard work. Think of what you're going to achieve! It's important to actively work against sabotaging yourself.

Quote: 'Challenges are what make life interesting; overcoming them is what makes life meaningful.' (Joshua J. Marine)

Exercise:
- Go for a walk/run three times for a minimum of forty-five minutes, and do it faster this time.
- Do the forty-minute cardio workout the trainer gave you. Do it harder. Do it faster.
- Do the bum squeezes, tummy tucks, stair thingies and sit-ups every day.
- Do two other sessions of cardio, and do at least two to three weights sessions.
- Do a video class at home.

Motivation: Take that reward, you winner. You've worked hard, you deserve it. What did you choose: a weekend away, sky diving or horse riding? Don't forget to measure yourself!

Week Nine

Goal: Repeat after me: 'I am strong. I am healthy. I am loved. I am powerful. I am in control. I deserve the very best in life.

I eat well. I nurture myself. I exercise as often as I should. I am well on the way to having the life I have always dreamed of.' With these things in mind, let this month be the very best one you've had so far. Eat well, move more, drink less, think happy thoughts. Step outside your comfort zone and try something new, like a team sport, and have some fun! Everything is going to be OK.

Quote: 'The harder you work the luckier you get.' (Gary Player)

Exercise:
- Join and play a team sport – soccer, basketball, netball, etc; or hook up with someone to regularly play tennis or squash. This is called your leisure sport. Do it every week . . . for fun!
- Go for a walk/run three times for a minimum of forty-five minutes.
- Do the forty-minute cardio workout the trainer gave you.
- Do the bum squeezes, tummy tucks, stair thingies and sit-ups every day.
- Do two other sessions of cardio, and do at least two to three weights sessions.

Motivation: Go over this last week. Once again, circle every time you have 'treated' yourself or not made a very good food choice. If you are doing it once a day, it's too much. Try and limit your treats to perhaps one every couple of days. Are they really worth sabotaging your goal weight? Pick the times you will have something naughty, and lock it in as a reward so that you work hard and can then enjoy it, guilt-free.

Week Ten

Goal: Try on those skinny jeans again. You may be pleasantly surprised. You may be closer to fitting into them than you think. If you don't have any skinny jeans, buy a dress that's just a little bit too tight and focus your energy on fitting into it. Every little thing you do counts, so keep honest and keep moving.

Quote: 'Life is either a daring adventure or nothing.' (Helen Keller)

Exercise:
- Play your leisure sport for one hour (minimum).
- Go for a walk/run three times for a minimum of forty-five minutes.
- Do the forty-minute cardio workout the trainer gave you.
- Do the bum squeezes, tummy tucks, stair thingies and sit-ups every day.
- Do two other sessions of cardio, and least two to three weights sessions.

Motivation: Don't let small obstacles become your undoing. Persistence and perseverance will ensure you'll get there in the end – and stay there!

Week Eleven

Goal: How badly do you want to walk in a room and be the best looking girl there? How badly do you want to walk down a beach in a slinky white bikini? How badly do you want to bump into your old friends from school and have them declare they didn't recognise you? It could be you. If you make this week as good as it can be, it *will* be you.

Quote: The person at the top of the mountain didn't fall there.

Exercise:
- Play your leisure sport for one hour (minimum).
- Go for a walk/run three times for a minimum of forty-five minutes.
- Do the forty-minute cardio workout the trainer gave you.
- Do the bum squeezes, tummy tucks, stair thingies and sit-ups every day.
- Do two other sessions of cardio and do at least two to three weights sessions.

Motivation: You should be a dress size down by now. If not, don't give up; use your disappointment to fuel you towards having an even better week. We learn by making mistakes so be thankful for every step you take because you are closer then you think. Remember: take one step at a time. You *will* get there.

Week Twelve

Goal: Exercise should be a priority. Put it in your diary and do not give it up for anything. Push yourself ever further by embracing a weekend fun-run. On the food side of things, keep lots of fresh fruit handy. Think of this last week in The Alfalfa Zone as the first week of the rest of your healthy, new, fit and active life. And go and have the best week possible!

Quote: Every end is a new beginning.

Exercise:
- Sign up to do a fun run. Train for the event and do it.
- Play your leisure sport for one hour (minimum).
- Go for a walk/run, or do a cardio workout four times for a minimum of forty-five minutes.
- Do the bum squeezes, tummy tucks, stair thingies and sit-ups every day.
- Do another session of cardio and do at least two to three weights sessions.

Motivation: Go and measure yourself, you shrinking violet! Don't think about how far you have to go, congratulate yourself on how far you have come, and just keep going.

Remember, it doesn't stop here. Keep going! Just treat it as the thing you do. Time will pass and if you keep eating well and exercising, you will achieve your dream of being fit, healthy, energetic, athletic, positive, powerful and successful. And if all else fails: bluff it until you become it. Now go and be the best that you can be.

Recipes

AJ's Seafood Pizza

One pizza base (you can substitute with lavash, pita or Lebanese
    bread)
One cup of tomato paste
80 g low fat ricotta
1 tbsp chopped basil (you can buy it in tubes now)
1 tbsp chopped garlic (you can buy this in tubes now, too)
One handful of fresh, uncooked prawns (peeled)
One handful of marinara mix
Half a handful of scallops
Small piece of white fish, like barramundi
Small piece of Atlantic salmon
½ capsicum, sliced
⅓ onion, sliced
1 tomato, sliced
6 mushrooms, sliced
1 tsp capers
6 anchovies (drained of oil)
⅓ cup low fat mozzarella
Red wine (optional)

Spread the pizza base with tomato paste, ricotta cheese, garlic and
basil (you can mix it all up together if you like, and then spread it
on). Sprinkle the prawns, marinara mix, scallops, fish, capsicum,
onion, tomato, mushrooms, capers, anchovies and mozzarella over
the top. Cook in pre-heated oven at 220 degrees for approximately
25–30 minutes.

Serves 4.
Approx 15 g fat and 580 calories per serve.

Quick Stir Fry

400 g hokkein noodles
200 g fresh marinated tofu
200 g diced chicken breast or lean veal
1 clove garlic
1 red onion, sliced
1 red capsicum, sliced
10 mushrooms, sliced
1 carrot, sliced
15 snow peas
2 tbsp soy sauce
1 tbsp hoi sin sauce
1 tbsp honey
1 tsp sesame seeds

In a large non-stick wok or frying pan brown meat and set aside. Using meat juices left in pan, stir-fry the garlic, vegetables and sauces. When vegetables are almost cooked, add tofu and cook until heated through. Prepare hokkein noodles as per directions on pack (microwave, run under hot water, or soak in boiling water). Add noodles and meat and stir through other ingredients in pan for another two minutes. Serve with sprinkle of sesame seeds.

Serves 4.
12 g fat and 600 calories per serve.

Roasted Baby Vegetables

1 kg baby potatoes
300 g baby carrots
200 g baby turnips
200 g sweet potato
200 g baby parsnips
200 g baby beetroot
2 small red onions
1 tbsp seeded mustard
100 mL maple syrup
2 cloves garlic

Chop all vegetables into small chunks, except baby carrots and beetroot. Boil or microwave potato, carrots, turnips, parsnips, beetroot, and sweet potato until almost cooked. Drain. Put vegetables in deep baking dish. Combine mustard, garlic and maple syrup. Pour over vegetables. Bake in an oven at around 220°C, stirring occasionally until vegetables are soft and browned (about 20–30 mins).

Serves 6.
0.8 g fat and 350 calories per serve.

Yummy Banana Bread

1¼ cups of self-raising flour
1 teaspoon of cinnamon
1 tbsp low fat butter
½ cup Splenda (sugar substitute)
1 egg, beaten
¼ cup low fat milk
½ cup mashed banana
10 walnuts – lightly crushed
1 tbsp poppy seeds

Spray a loaf tin with cooking oil or line with baking paper. Mix flour and cinnamon in a bowl, and rub in butter. Stir in Splenda, egg, milk, banana, walnuts and poppy seeds.

Pour into loaf pan and bake for about 20 minutes at 220°C. **Note:** I often double the mix (and cook for longer) and add blueberries or strawberries to taste.

Makes 1 loaf (serves 6).
4 g fat and 300 calories per serve (2 slices).

Bagel Chips

2 wholemeal bagels
Olive oil or canola cooking spray
1 clove of garlic, crushed
2 tbsp tandoori paste
2 tbsp horseradish cream

Cut whole bagels into very thin slices and arrange on an oven tray in single layer. Spray lightly with cooking oil. Scatter crushed garlic over bagel slices. Brush tandoori paste over half, and horseradish cream over the other half. Bake in oven at 220°C for 15 minutes until brown and crisp. Serve with hommous or beetroot dip.

Makes about 16 bagel chips.
Approximately 4 g fat and 150 calories per bagel chip.

Quickie Potato Bake

Use one large washed potato per person. Stab potato five or six times with a skewer and cook in microwave for about six minutes, or until soft. Cut open at the top and sprinkle a mix of sun-dried tomato, fat-free bacon or ham, mushrooms, onion and low fat cheese on top. Bake in oven at 220°C for about ten minutes, until other ingredients have heated through and cheese has melted.

Approximately 7 g fat and 360 calories per serve.

Ham and Mushroom Omelette

4 eggs, beaten lightly
6 egg whites (extra)
450 g mushrooms
200 g low fat or lite ham
¼ cup parsley, finely chopped
¼ cup grated low fat cheese

Combine beaten egg and extra egg whites in a bowl. Beat well. Cook mushrooms in a non-stick frypan, adding ham at the last minute to heat through. Take off heat and stir through parsley. Pour a quarter of egg mixture into non-stick frypan on low heat. Cook till almost done. Spoon a quarter of mushroom and ham mixture on the top of the omelette, and sprinkle over cheese. Fold over half of omelette and heat until cheese melts. Slide onto plate and serve. Repeat three more times.

Serves 4.
6 g fat and 320 calories per serve.

Spaghetti Bolognaise

1 small brown onion, chopped
2 cloves garlic, chopped finely
2 small carrots, chopped
2 zucchinis, chopped
5 medium mushrooms, sliced
400 g lean mince (beef)
2 cups tomato pasta sauce
400 g tin Italian tomatoes, chopped
½ cup veggie stock
1 cup red wine (optional; use more if you feel the urge)
2 bay leaves
500 g packet spaghetti

Cook onion and garlic in non-stick frypan until soft. Add carrots, zucchinis and mushrooms and cook until soft. Add beef and cook until it browns. Add pasta sauce, wine, tomatoes, stock and bay leaves. Bring to the boil then reduce heat and simmer for about fifteen to twenty minutes. Cook pasta (approximately 100 g dry spaghetti per person) until al dente, serve in bowls and spoon over bolognaise sauce. **Note:** This tastes even better the next day or night as the flavours deepen.

Serves 4.
12 g fat and 600 calories per serve.

Sweet Potato and Corn Frittata

1 sweet potato
1 small tin corn kernels
1 brown onion
6 mushrooms
1 tbsp raw sugar
4 eggs
3 egg whites (extra)
½ cup low fat milk
½ cup low fat cheddar (grated)
Olive oil or canola cooking spray

Chop sweet potato into 2 cm cubes. Toss sweet potato, onion and sugar together and place on baking tray. Spray lightly with cooking spray. Bake for 30 minutes in a hot oven, until potato is golden brown. Cook mushrooms in non-stick frypan. Beat eggs and egg whites separately. Combine all ingredients in bowl and mix well. Line baking dish with baking paper and pour in combined ingredients. Bake in an oven at 220°C for 35 minutes. Cut into squares and serve with salad.

Serves 4.
Approximately 9 g fat and 310 calories per serve.

Honeyed Chicken Breast

1 chicken breast (no skin)
2 tbsp honey
2 tbsp white vinegar
2 tbsp seeded mustard
2 tsp soy sauce

Marinate chicken in all other ingredients for at least 3 hours (overnight is best). Cook in baking dish, uncovered, in an oven at 220°C for approximately 15–20 minutes, or until chicken breast is tender and moist. Serve breast with juice from baking dish and accompany with salad.

Serves 1.
9 g fat and 450 calories per serve.

Yummy Fish for Two

2 fillets of white fish (I prefer barramundi or flathead)
2 tbsp fresh ginger
2 cloves garlic
1 tbsp soy sauce
1 tbsp hoi sin sauce
1 tbsp sherry
1 tbsp brown sugar
¼ cup veggie stock
Shallots, chopped

Line tray with piece of foil long enough to fold over. Place fish fillets on foil. Mix ingredients in a small bowl and pour over fish. Pinch foil together to make a parcel and bake in an oven at 220°C for about fifteen minutes or until cooked through. Place fish on plate and drizzle with sauce from foil. Serve with salad or rice and steamed vegies.

Serves 2.
9 g fat and 350 calories per serve.

Tuna and Spinach Lasagne

4 mushrooms, sliced finely
1 clove of garlic, crushed
1 onion, sliced
425 g tuna in spring water, drained
325g canned, chopped tomatoes
1 cup tomato puree
1 lemon
250 g packet frozen spinach
½ cup basil leaves, shredded
100 g low fat ricotta
400 g packet lasagne sheets
½ cup breadcrumbs
½ cup low fat grated cheese
Olive or canola oil cooking spray

Preheat oven to 210°C. Spray a saucepan with cooking oil. Cook onion until soft and then add garlic, mushroom, tuna, tomatoes, half the puree, basil and lemon juice. Cook until mushroom is cooked through. Mix through ricotta. Spoon ¼ cup of remaining puree into bottom of baking dish. Layer with lasagne sheets, then ½ tuna mix, another layer of lasagne sheets, then layer with remaining tuna mix. Top with final layer of lasagne sheets. Spoon last of puree over the top and sprinkle with breadcrumbs and cheese. Bake for approximately 35 minutes.

Serves 6.
10 g fat and 500 calories per serve.

Quick Fish

One fillet of Atlantic salmon
½ lemon
¼ lime
Fresh dill, chopped
Fresh parsley, chopped
½ clove of garlic, crushed

Place fish fillet on foil on baking tray. Squeeze lemon and lime over fish. Add garlic, parsley, and dill. Pinch foil together to make a parcel and bake for 10–15 minutes in an oven at 220°C, or until fish is cooked.

Serves 1.
10 g fat and 320 calories per serve.

Smoked Salmon Pancakes

Olive or canola oil cooking spray
1 cup white self-raising flour
1 egg
1 cup low fat milk
salt
250 g smoked salmon
¼ Attiki Natural low fat yoghurt
1 bunch chives
1 tsp fresh dill, chopped finely
2 tbsp capers, chopped finely

These are excellent for parties! Combine egg, flour, milk and pinch of salt and beat well.

Spray frypan lightly with cooking oil. Heat pan on medium heat. Pour in mixture to make small pancakes. When bubbles appear throughout pancake, flip and cook through. Cool on wire rack. Shred smoked salmon and mix through yoghurt. Mix capers, lemon juice, dill and chives together separately. On each pancake spoon one quantity of smoked salmon mixture and garnish with small dollop of caper mix. Enjoy but don't eat too many!

Makes about 20 pancakes.
0.5 g fat and 35 calories per serve.

Spinach and Mushroom Risotto with Pine Nuts

1 onion, chopped
1 clove garlic, crushed
1 cup of mixed mushrooms, sliced
1 cup of raw risotto rice (e.g arborio)
3½ cups low fat veggie stock
100 g baby spinach leaves
fresh rosemary, chopped
cracked pepper
1 tbsp parmesan cheese
2 tbsp roasted pine nuts
Olive or canola oil cooking spray

Spray saucepan with oil and cook garlic and onion until soft. Add mushrooms, rosemary and rice, then one cup of stock. Stir until rice has absorbed the stock. Slowly add more stock, stirring continuously, until rice has absorbed all liquid (rice will be soft and creamy). Take off heat, stir through baby spinach leaves, add cracked pepper to taste, and shredded parmesan. Sprinkle with pine nuts.

Serves 4.
7 grams fat and 270 calories per serve.

Mixed Berry Pancakes

1 cup self-raising flour
1 tsp baking powder
300 g low fat French vanilla Vaalia yoghurt
4 egg whites
4 egg yolks
2 tbsp blueberries
1 punnet strawberries
2 tbsp raspberries
Maple syrup
Olive or canola cooking spray

Sift flour and baking powder in bowl. Add egg yolks and yoghurt and stir until combined.

Beat egg whites until soft peaks form. Fold egg whites through batter, being careful not to overmix. Heat large frypan and spray lightly with oil. Pour in batter to preferred size of pancake, cook until bubbles appear, flip and cook again until firm. Keep cooked pancakes on plate and cover in foil to keep warm. Serve with berries and maple syrup.

Serves 4.
3.5 g fat and 200 calories per serve.

Tiramisu

3 eggs
¼ cup caster sugar
¼ cup white self-raising flour
¼ cup wholemeal self-raising flour
¼ cup cornflour
1 teaspoon gelatine
1 tablespoon cold water
320 g low fat ricotta
¼ cup low fat milk
¼ cup quality, plungered, chocolate coffee (e.g. Gloria Jeans
    Mudslide)
⅓ cup low fat milk
½ cup Kahlua
25 g Flake Noir (dark chocolate bar)
6 strawberries, halved

This recipe is best cooked the day before you need it. Preheat oven to 220°C. Grease and line a spring-loaded round cooking tin. Sift the three flours twice (into one bowl). Discard wheat husks and set flour aside. Beat eggs well until thick and creamy. Add ½ cup sugar and mix until dissolved. Gently fold in sifted flour and mix until combined. Pour into tin and bake for about 25 minutes. Allow cake to cool on wire tray.

Pour cold water into (heatproof) plastic or glass measuring cup. Sprinkle gelatine over water. Place cup in small saucepan filled with simmering water, or cook in microwave, stirring frequently until gelatine is dissolved. Allow to cool. Using a blender, mix ricotta, milk and remaining sugar (¼ cup). Add gelatine and mix through until creamy.

Make plunger coffee and add Kahlua and milk. Cut cake in half horizontally. Place half in spring-loaded tin, and put tin on a plate.

Lightly drizzle half of coffee mixture over cake so that it is fully covered. Use a pastry brush to even it out, making sure cake is well moistened. Add half of ricotta mixture. Place other half of sponge on top. Drizzle remaining coffee mixture over cake. Add remaining ricotta mixture on top.

Refrigerate for at least four hours. Release from tin and crumble flake chocolate over cake and decorate with strawberries.

Enjoy but make sure you don't have seconds!

Serves 8.
6 grams of fat and 210 calories per serve.
Cut slices smaller if you want to reduce your fat and calorie intake.

Q & A

Here are some of the most common questions I'm asked at the Healthy Body Club.

Q: **Why poached eggs over fried?**
A: Poaching your eggs is the best option because there is no oil used in the cooking process. It's pretty failsafe when you're ordering breakfast at a café. However, at home, where you can control the cooking process, you can use a non-stick pan and 'fry' your eggs instead, if you prefer. Poaching doesn't reduce the fat in the egg itself but it does ensure there's none extra used.

Q: **Why is alcohol bad for weight loss?**
A: Alcohol has what is termed 'empty calories'. This means the calories in alcohol have no nutritional value whatsoever. Also, when you drink alcohol everything else your body is metabolising gets put on hold until the alcohol is 'dealt with' i.e. broken down and got rid of. So the food you eat while you're drinking just sits there. While the liver is processing the alcohol, your food isn't being dealt with as it normally would be when you aren't drinking, and no fat gets burned from your body.

On top of this you're more likely to eat junk food, or make unhealthy food choices, because alcohol increases your appetite and decreases your ability to say 'no'. If you add a hangover to the whole thing you could lose one to two days of burning fat. It's best just to take it easy, or abstain altogether if you can. I find I can lose between two and three kilos in a month by changing nothing else but my alcohol intake.

Q: **What is the difference between skim, lite and Shape milk? What is better?**

A: All of these are good choices as they are all low in fat. Basically skim milk is termed as a 'no fat' milk because the amount of fat it has in it is negligible; Shape is also a 'no fat' milk, but with added calcium; and Lite milk is a reduced fat milk. For the least fatty intake from your milk, skim and Shape are the ones to choose. However, for women I particularly recommend any 'no fat' or light milk that has added calcium (like Shape). We need calcium for strong bones and teeth, which will help us to avoid osteoporosis in later life.

Q: **When buying food do I get the lowest in fat or in sugar?**

A: Choosing low in fat is better. Sugars get converted into energy and have a window of time in which they can be burned off (after that it gets turned into fat). However, fat remains as it is and is stored as fat. Keep in mind, though, that 50 extra unburned calories a day can add up to a 2 kg increase in a year so it's good to try and keep your sugar content down as well.

Q: **What's the difference between a calorie and a kilojoule?**

A: They are one and the same: they're both units of measurement of the energy values in food (which roughly translates as a measurement of sugars and carbohydrates in food). If this is confusing, think of calories as miles and kilojoules as kilometres. One calorie is equivalent to 4.186 kilojoules, so if you need to convert kilojoules to calories, just divide the kilojoule figure by 4.186 and you'll have your calorie value. Kilojoules are not four times as fattening as calories – they're both just units of measurements.

Q: **When cooking with wine does it still keep its calorie content?**

A: Yes, it does, unfortunately. Try using only a little bit of wine and using veggie stock as a substitute for the liquid instead.

Q: **What bread is better for me? White, brown, wholegrain, packet bread or fresh bread from the baker's?**

A: Well, brown bread is actually higher in the GI than white (yes, it's true). However, wholegrain is best all round in terms of low GI and its nutrient levels. Bread from the baker is usually higher in sugar but some offer low fat, no sugar versions. Sourdough is an excellent, low GI choice when buying fresh bread.

Q: **How do I cook food without too much oil?**

A: Use cooking oil spray, stocks, water, lemon juice or vinegar. Cook meat slowly to allow its juices to come out and aid in the cooking. Cook veggies in the microwave, or steam them in a steamer; or, using a pastry brush, brush lightly with oil and crisp under the griller.

Q: **I don't want to make one meal for me and another for my family. What should I do?**

A: Learn to cook low fat food for the entire family. Kids can eat low fat food from age two and a half. By age five they should be eating low fat food anyway. They might say they don't like it but if you get some good recipe books they won't know the difference at all. The starving children in Ethiopia don't turn down food because they don't like the taste. Also, if your family is hungry enough they will eat what you serve up. Whatever you do, don't make your kids fat as well. Start living healthily as a family *now*.

Q: I eat fairly healthy snacks but when I open a packet of lollies or pretzels, I end up eating the whole packet. What can I do to stop this?

A: Portion control was one of the toughest things I had to deal with. Avoid relying on willpower – it doesn't exist. I break packets of lollies and pretzels into small plastic bags in the right serving size. Those re-sealable plastic bags do the trick very well. Keep them at the back of your pantry or fridge – out of sight is out of mind.

Q: I am so busy I never have time to eat well and can only ever get McDonald's. How can I stop this?

A: Be a good girl guide and be prepared. Take food with you – everywhere. It takes less time to make and take a sandwich than it does to go to the take-away shop, line up, order, wait for and then eat something that will do you no good. Make a double serving of stir-fry for dinner, portion it up and take it to work the next day. Reheating takes two minutes and you don't even have to leave the office. Before you walk out the door, have a guestimate of how long you will be gone for and take enough food or snacks to get you through.

Q: If I am counting my calories and the only dinner option is to have something that is 200 calories more should I just skip the meal until I can eat something else?

A: No, never skip meals. You'll only tell your body to go
into fat storage mode. If the food is 200 calories, just eat
half of it. Or, if you do eat the whole lot, go for a walk to
burn the extra calories off. There will be days when you
will have more calories than others and counting calories is no way to live your life. I only ever guessed at my
calorie intake. I was never very strict except when I hit a
plateau. The idea is to make the best choices possible
and enjoy your treats when you have them.

Q: **There is a lot of talk about 'good fats'. Does this mean
I can have a lot of them?**

A: Fat gets stored as fat. Even good fats eaten to excess get
stored as fat and *will* interfere or halt your weight loss.
You'd be amazed how only a few 'healthy' (or 'good fat')
nuts can add up to one single day's intake of fat. If you
do decide to eat good fats, like avocado, almonds etc,
keep an eye on how much you're eating, making sure
that it doesn't blow your day's intake in one hit.

Q: **I have never eaten breakfast and not only don't feel
hungry but often feel ill at the mere thought of food.
Can't I just wait until morning tea to eat?**

A: Nope. You can't skip breakfast. It's one of the very few
rules you can't break if you want to lose weight and keep
it off. The moment you eat, you kickstart your metabolism and start burning fat. The reason why you aren't
hungry is because your metabolism has ground to a
standstill. When you wake up, your last meal was probably over fourteen hours ago (at dinner time the night
before) and your body needs to know it's being fed so
that it can start burning fat again. If you start eating
breakfast, within the first two weeks of doing so, you will

begin to wake up feeling hungry and sometimes be so ravenous the first thing you do is eat. That is the sign of a healthy metabolism.

Q: How do I keep my kids treats in the cupboard without me pigging out on them?

A: You don't. Why give your kids food that they will only have to work off later in life? Give your children the best opportunity to live a normal, healthy life. Obesity is the fastest growing epidemic in Australia. Teach them to eat healthy snacks. Red licorice and jelly snakes are better choices than chips or chocolate. Sure, they should be able to have the odd bit of junk food but leave it for when you're out; not at home. If you're determined to keep treats at home, just buy them stuff they love but which you are not so keen on. The reality is that they should be snacking mostly on fruit.

Q: I've heard that you should not eat in the morning before a workout. Will that help me lose weight faster?

A: Always eat breakfast. I totally disagree with this theory of skipping food before a morning workout. It has been too long since you have eaten last. You need energy to get through the exercise. Yes, you will lose weight if you don't eat but when the body is not fed the first thing it does is eat muscle so you just undo all the good work you have done in the gym. Don't send your body into starvation mode. Just eat lightly; have a banana and a glass of milk if you want to limit your food and have something more substantial after your workout. Regular meals and exercise teach the body to burn excess fat. I lost over forty kilos without skipping any meals. You can too.

Q: Should I wait an hour after a workout before eating food?

A: Some experts say yes and some say no. I found it so confusing. The reality is that after a workout you need protein to repair and grow muscle; and if you are hungry or if it is snack time you should eat. You don't want your body going into starvation mode. If you are so hungry that you start fantasising about food you are more likely to have a breakout so control those cravings and feed your body the fuel it needs. Just make a healthy choice.

Q: Can I eat as much as I like as long as it is low fat?

A: No. Weight loss is a simple equation: input versus output. If you overeat *anything* you are consuming excess calories and fat, and you will put on weight.

Contacts and Services

Health

Australian Government and State contacts

Australian Government Department of Health and Ageing:
www.health.gov.au

Australian Capital Territory Department of Health:
www.health.act.gov.au

Indigenous health support: www.healthinfonet.ecu.edu.au

New South Wales Government Department of Health:
www.health.nsw.gov.au

Northern Territory Government Department of Health:
www.health.nt.gov.au

Queensland Government Department of Health:
www.health.qld.gov.au

South Australian Government Department of Health:
www.dhs.sa.gov.au

Tasmanian Government Department of Health:
www.dhhs.tas.gov.au

Victorian Government Department of Health: www.better
health.vic.gov.au

Western Australian Government Department of Health:
www.health.wa.gov.au

Children's health

Children's health development foundation:
www.chdf.org.au

Childhood obesity:
www.medicineau.net.au/clinical/obesity/obesit1275.html

Eating disorders and mental health

Eating Disorders Foundation: www.eatingdisorders.org.au;
NSW: (02) 9412 4499, VIC: (03) 9885 0318, QLD: (07)
3876 2500, SA: (08) 8212 1644

NSW Eating Disorders Support and Info (02) 9412 4499

Tasmanian Community Nutrition Unit (03) 6222 7222

WA Eating Disorders Centre (08) 9335 1440

New Zealand Eating Disorders Association Inc:
www.health.auckland.ac.nz/community/community_gro
ups/eda.html

Overeaters Anonymous: www.overeatersanonymous.org

ACT Mental Health ACT 1800 629 354

NT Association for Mental Health (08) 8981 4128

Anxiety Disorders Alliance freecall 1800 626 055 or
(02) 9570 4519

Help lines

Lifeline: 131 114

Kids Help Line: 1800 55 800

Distress Call Christian Help Line: 1300 364 454

Sporting organisations

National

Australian Government Sports Commission:
www.ausport.gov.au

State by State

ACT: www.sport.act.gov.au

NSW: www.sportnsw.com.au, www.dsr.nsw.gov.au

NT: www.dcdsca.nt.gov.au

QLD: www.sportrec.qld.gov.au
SA: www.recsport.sa.gov.au, www.sportsa.org.au
TAS: www.osr.tas.gov.au
VIC: www.sport.vic.gov.au
WA: www.dsr.wa.gov.au

Women's sport
Womensport: www.womensport.com.au

Soccer
Australian Soccer: www.australiansoccer.com.au

Running
Fun run information: www.coolrunning.com.au
The City to Surf: www.sunherald.com.au/city2surf
Asics Walk for Wellbeing:
    www.femail.com.au/asics_walk_for_wellbeing.htm
Nike Women's Classic: www.eventwizard.com.au

Health, fitness and weight loss support services

Fernwood Women's Health Club: www.fernwood.net.au
Healthy Body Club (AJ Rochester):
    www.healthybodyclub.com.au
The Health Fitness Directory, by Stefan Angheli:
    www.healthfitness.com.au
Weight Watchers Australia: www.weightwatchers.com.au

Family support

Parents Without Partners: <u>www.pwp.org.au</u>
Lone Parent Family Support Service (NSW):
   (02) 9251 5622

Thank Youse

My darling boy, Kai. I love you with all my heart and soul. It is so nice to see you happy and finding your spirit again.

Crusher for showing me the truth, the weigh and the lite. Amen!

Dr Nutcase for continuing to keep me sane. You have no idea how grateful I am to you. You help me totally transform my life on a daily basis.

Roberta Ivers, my editor – honestly, without you this book would not be a reality. You should have a credit on the cover, you did so much. I don't know how you do what you do – even I can't make sense of my waffle sometimes and you just seem to know what I mean. But you are more than that – a buddy, a soccer mate, a confidante, a career advisor and a friend.

Selwa Anthony, my agent, who made my writing career a reality and continues to do so.

Fiona Henderson, my publisher, for believing in me once again.

Mia Freedman – your support, both professionally and personally, helped me through one of the toughest times of my life. Thank you for paving the way for the anti-diet revolution. Thank you for helping women empower and love themselves. Thank you for showing the world there is something other than a size 10 woman and that she is a beautiful thing. Thank you for doing all you have to help me. I am truly, truly grateful.

Ros Gibson – you are the closest I have to a mum. You make me feel like someone cares about me on a day-to-day basis. You are an inspiration.

Zoë Williams – you are always so positive about everything. Thank you for always being there, and for all your fantastic input, your encouraging words. Thank you for being my best friend, my mother, my sister, my brother; sometimes you are even more of a boyfriend than my boyfriends. I love you (particularly for cleaning the house around me while I write this).

Minna – thanks for being such a great big sister to Kai and such a wonderful little sister to me.

Ziggy – thanks for being such a good 'big brother' to Kai.

Leash – I can never repay you for all that you do for Kai and me. Choosing you to be his godmother was the smartest decision I have ever made. Thank you from the heart of my bottom. And the same goes to you Aunty Allison, we love you too.

Jussy (aka Karen) Biddlestix – you are a true friend. You are such a beautiful person, loyal and devoted.

Thanks to Richie for designing the best website ever (http://www.webstudio-1.com.au/).

Paul Mudgway (p.mudgway@optusnet.com.au) for the fabulous logo for my Healthy Body Club.

Tara, Dannan and Daniel for always being there for Kai.

Jules – mwah mwah mwah, sweetie darling. Thanks for all the support.

Claire (chocolatey) – looking forward to a long friendship with you, babe. Thank you for all you have done for me.

Moony for your friendship and support when I needed it most.

Scott, my soccer coach for making me less of a Blubberguts and more Beckham-like (I wish). You have taught me so much. Thank you for taking the time and effort to teach me all the little things that make my game even more enjoyable.

Thomas Gray, my English and Drama teacher when I was sixteen, for taking time out of your lunch-hour to have a quick conversation that literally changed the course of my life.

Gary Whale for continuing to inspire me and for still taking the time to make me feel special.

Allison Brennan at Random House, for being the best publicist in the whole world. Thanks heaps, mate! Love your work!

Suzy and Kathy at Fernwood Broadway for all their support.

All my girls from The 5 Kilo Club.

Every single person who wrote to me. Thank you for sharing your stories with me. I wouldn't have written this if you hadn't asked me to.

To everyone who has helped me through some of my darkest times.

And last but not least . . . thank you to the universe (God) for always protecting and guiding me.

Go Tigers and go Man U!

Index

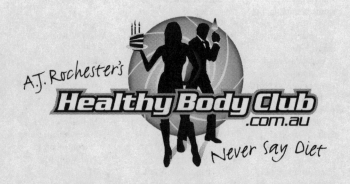

A.J. Rochester's

Healthy Body Club
.com.au

Never Say Diet